TECHNOLOGY AND MEDICINE

Taking a holistic approach, this book describes the developments in medicine and medical technology from ancient times to modern days. It is an exciting journey where the readers will learn about the many great inventions by people that did not take the knowledge of their times as a fact. They challenged mysticism, beliefs, religion, and the Church. They were true scientists long before we knew how to define what a scientist is. This book is, in a way, connecting the dots between the past and the future within healthcare.

Features

- Provides details on further developments that gave new and exceptional information for diagnostic or therapeutic purposes
- Gives the reader a new perspective and a common thread of life on medicine and MedTech as well as an improved understanding of how far we have come and how much there still is to work on before we fully understand the human body and its functionality
- Discusses and gives insight into ongoing research projects that could become clinically available in the future

Bengt Nielsen is CEO of nielseninnovation AB and holds a PhD in radiation physics. He has been a hospital physicist in radiology for 11 years and spent 25 years at GE HealthCare in different international leadership positions, primarily within marketing and medical research. Today, his work is mainly focused on supporting medical start-up businesses to reach the market and to obtain a clinical introduction, lecturing at the Senior University in Stockholm, and participating in expert groups validating research grant applications primarily from Scandinavian researchers.

T0260385

TECHNOLOGY AND MEDICINE

Shaping Modern Healthcare

Bengt Nielsen

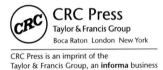

CRC Press
Taylor & Francis Group
Boca Raton London New York

CRC Press is an imprint of the
Taylor & Francis Group, an **informa** business

First edition published 2024
by CRC Press
6000 Broken Sound Parkway NW, Suite 300, Boca Raton, FL 33487–2742

and by CRC Press
4 Park Square, Milton Park, Abingdon, Oxon, OX14 4RN

CRC Press is an imprint of Taylor & Francis Group, LLC

ISBN: 978-1-032-49340-4 (hbk)
ISBN: 978-1-032-49337-4 (pbk)
ISBN: 978-1-003-39332-0 (ebk)

DOI: 10.1201/9781003393320

Typeset in New Baskerville Std
by Apex CoVantage, LLC

CONTENTS

ACKNOWLEDGMENTS

Writing a book takes time, and it is a real stretch, as it needs your concentration and endurance over a long period. Many of the things that needs to be done on our real estate have been postponed or have just not been done for a long time.

In spite of the challenges, I do not regret that I started this project. I think my endurance and curiosity helped me through the many days, including the late nights.

Writing is also a lonely occupation. It would not work for me without support from someone. My dear wife, Kerstin, has always supported me when I needed it the most. During the more than two years that this book project has taken, she has been an outstanding support. On top of taking the full responsibility for everything in our daily life, she has seen to it that I got food, drink, sleep, and very importantly, exercise and fresh air every day. Without Kerstin, this project would not have been finished and my many references would not have been in the right place and in the right order. It is hard to find the right way to credit her.

Maybe it is to promise her not to write another book. Honestly, I am not ready yet to make such a tough promise. (Between you and me, I have an idea.)

There are several other people to whom I am very grateful that have had different roles during my lifetime. Our four children, Anna, Fredrik, Åsa, and Claes, have always been encouraging, positive, and helpful.

When I reflect back, there are also persons that have meant a lot to me but that are not with us anymore, like my late mother, Ester, and late nanny, Gunbritt Persson, who encouraged and led me to higher education when I was too young to understand the importance of education.

The many excellent and brilliant people whom I have had the pleasure to work with and who gave me the insight into new, exciting things through my working life. I can only mention some of them who stick out. Leonard Fass, PhD; Oncology Professor Gordon McVie; Cardiology Professor Mattias Fredrich; Felix Wehrli, PhD, Professor of Radiologic Science; Chief Radiologist and Neuroradiologists Claes Rådberg and Inge-Gerd Johansson; late Professor of Radiology Paul Edholm; Lead Engineer Viggo Fransson; late Professor Carl Carlsson; Professor Emerita Gudrun Alm Carlsson;

Professor Emeritus Bengt Långström; Radiologist Mike Bourne; Former Vice President of Sales at GE HealthCare Jean Yves Burel and Vice President of Business Operations Mohamed Ababsa.

I want to thank you all from the bottom of my heart, for your encouragement, leadership, and support. Some of you know what you mean for me, while some of you may be surprised, as you acted a bit in the background, but your leadership and teaching style stimulated me tremendously. I am very grateful for your always kind, candid, and gentle teaching style.

Many thanks to all of you for having made my very intense working period such a joyful experience.

I am rather sure I have missed mentioning several of the fantastic teachers and mentors from my very joyful career. My sincere apologies. Many thanks to all of you for giving me the well-needed encouragement to learn many new things, including things a bit out my comfort zone.

Finally, I want to thank the people at my publisher, CRC Press/Taylor & Francis, especially my medical editor, Shivangi Pramanik, who believed in me and my topic and saw to it that I got an agreement with Taylor & Francis.

Lastly, I want to thank Himani Dwivedi and Jacob Jewitt-Jallan at CRC Press/Taylor & Francis for their patience and guidance in getting the manuscript in shape. It must have been tough to work with somebody just entering the very steep learning curve of how to publish a book. In my defense, I can only say that next time, it will be less stressful for all of you. I have learned a lot during this process.

To cite a former colleague from Linköping University, "Nothing is useless to a poet." I did not understand the real meaning before, now, I think I do.

Bengt Nielsen

INTERESTING AND STIMULATING READINGS

1. Yuval Noah Harari. *Sapiens, A Brief History of Mankind.* Leonhardt & Höier Literary Agency, Copenhagen. 2012.
2. Lindsey Fitzharris. *The Butchering Art: Joseph Lister's Quest to Transform the Grisly World of Victorian Medicine.* Published by arrangement with Scientific American Farrar, Straus and Giroux, New York. 2017.
3. Walter Isaacson. *Leonardo da Vinci.* Atlantis, Stockholm. 2017.
4. Toni Mount. *Medieval Medicine. Its Mysteries and Science.* Amberly Publishing, The Hill, Stroud Gloucestershire. 2015.
5. Hans Rosling, Anna Rosling Rönnlund, and Ola Rosling. *Factfullness.* Natur & Kultur, 2018. In Swedish.
6. *The Britannica Guide to the 100 Most Influential Scientists.* Introduction by John Gribbin. Robinson, an imprint of Constable & Robinson. 2008.
7. Sanjey Gupta. *Keep Sharp: Build a Better Brain at Any Age.* Simon & Schuster. 2021.
8. Svante Pääbo. *The Neanderthal Homo.* Fri Tanke Förlag. 2014. In Swedish.
9. Larry Scheckel. *Ask a Science Teacher: 250 Answers to Questions You've Always Had about How Everyday Stuff Really Works.* Workman Publishing Company Inc. 2013.
10. Kaja Nordengren. *The Brain Is the Star (Hjärnan är Stjärnan).* In Swedish. Kagge Förlag, in agreement with Stilton Literary Agency. 2016. Introduction by May-Britt Moser, Nobel Laureate.
11. Gerd Rosenbusch, Annemarie de Knecht-van Eekelen. *Wilhelm Conrad Röntgen: The Birth of Radiology.* Springer Biographies, 2019.
12. Harper, R. F. (2013). *The Code of Hammurabi, King of Babylon: About 2250 B.C.* CreateSpace Independent Publishing Platform.
13. Geller, M. J. (2010). *Ancient Babylonian Medicine: Theory and Practice.* Chichester, West Sussex, UK: Wiley-Blackwell.
14. Oppenheim, A. L., & Reiner, E. (1977). *Ancient Mesopotamia: Portrait of a Dead Civilization.* Chicago: University of Chicago Press.
15. Biggs, R. D. (2005). "Medicine, Surgery, and Public Health in Ancient Mesopotamia." *Journal of Assyrian Academic Studies.*
16. Horstmanshoff, H. F. L., Stol, M., & Tilburg, C. R. (2004). *Magic and Rationality in Ancient Near Eastern and Graeco-Roman Medicine.* Leiden: Brill.

PREFACE

How It All Started

Let's begin with some definitions:

> *Medicine* is the *art*, *science*, and *practice* of caring for a patient and managing the diagnosis, prognosis, prevention, treatment, or palliation of their injury or disease.
>
> *Science* (from the Latin word *scientia*, meaning "knowledge") is a systematic enterprise that builds and organizes knowledge in the form of testable explanations and predictions about the universe.
>
> *MedTech* is *products*, *techniques*, and *methods* that are used for treatment, medical care, diagnosis, and improvement or keeping of our health.

- It can be advanced equipment in hospitals or products that we are using in our homes.
- More advanced techniques, like X-ray units, CT scanners, MRI units, together with radiotherapy apparatus, orthopedic implants, stents, scalpels, IT and medical records systems, e-health solutions, walkers, pacemakers, dialysis machines, and so on, are mostly to be found at hospitals or medical clinics.

The earliest roots of science in medicine and healthcare can be traced to ancient Egypt and Mesopotamia from around 3500 BC to 3000 BC. Their contributions to mathematics, astronomy, and medicine also shaped the Greek natural philosophy of classical antiquity, whereby formal attempts were made to provide explanations of events in the physical world based on natural causes. Medicine encompasses a variety of healthcare practices evolved to maintain and restore health through the prevention and treatment of illnesses. Today's medicine applies biomedical sciences, biomedical research, genetics, and medical technology to diagnose, treat, and prevent injury and disease, typically through pharmaceuticals or surgery but also through therapies as diverse as psychotherapy, medical devices, biology, ionizing radiation, and so on.[1]

Medicine has been practiced since prehistoric times and was based on very few facts and knowledge. Frequently, the practice had connections to religious and philosophical beliefs and local culture. For example, a medicine

man would apply herbs and say prayers for healing or an ancient philosopher and physician would apply bloodletting according to the theories of
humorism (see Section 2.1 for definition).

In recent centuries, since the advent of modern science, most medicine
has become a combination of art and science (both basic and applied, under
the umbrella of medical science). While stitching technique for sutures is an
art learned through practice, the knowledge of what happens at the cellular
and molecular level in the tissues being stitched arises through science.

Pre-scientific forms of medicine are now known as *traditional medicine*
and *folk medicine*. They remain commonly used with, or instead of, scientific medicine and are, thus, called *alternative medicine*. For example, evidence on the effectiveness of acupuncture is variable and inconsistent for
any condition but is generally safe when done by an appropriately trained
practitioner.

In contrast, *alternative treatments* outside the bounds not just of scientific medicine but also of safety and efficacy are termed *quackery*. This can
encompass an array of practices and practitioners, irrespective of whether
they are pre-scientific (traditional medicine and folk medicine) or modern
pseudoscientific, including chiropractic, which rejects modern scientific
germ theory of disease and/or the science of immunization. Instead, they
believe without evidence that human diseases are caused by invisible sub-
luxation of the bones, predominantly of the spine and less so of other
bones.

Due to advances in medicine and MedTech, we can now treat many of the
diseases that formerly would have been fatal for the patient. Understanding
the advances that have occurred since primitive mankind and the challenges
that went along with the discoveries can help us appreciate the advances in
healthcare over the past 5000 years.[1]

Early in Our History

- We were superstitious and believed in witch doctors.
- We used herbs and plants as medicines. In fact, some of these are still
  used today.

Medicine comprises everything that we need during our lifetime. No wonder
this field has created so much interest in mankind and continues to engage
every living human.

The continued scientific developments through the centuries have had
a major impact on the lifetime of most humans around the world. The
expected lifetime for the Egyptians 5,000 years ago was 25–35 years. Today,
we have an expected lifetime of close to 100 years. In fact, the increased
lifetime of today tells us that most probably, some of the babies born today
could very well reach 130 years of age.[1]

Let Me Tell You a Little Personal Anecdote

During a yearly symposium on healthcare that was organized by *The Economist* and that took place around 2010 in Geneva, Switzerland, the introductory lecture was around the increased life expectance created by our improved healthcare systems. The lecturer told us that we could expect the lifetime to reach 128 years within 10 to 15 years. Close to 12 years have passed now since this lecture, and I am not sure if we already have reached the age of 128 yet, but we are probably not far from it today. I read recently that the oldest person in the world recently died at the age of 122 years.

After the talk, and the presentation was open for discussion, a gentleman from a European country stood up and looked rather desperate. His exact words, I cannot remember, but the essence was clear. He desperately expressed his concern for his country: "Our pension system is not able to handle this rapid increase of life expectancy. Please don't do this to us we cannot afford it!"

This person pointed at an important perspective of the fact that we live longer and longer, even if his reaction was both comic and tragic at the same time.

We all want to live longer with optimal life quality, but it will demand new developments within our society for individuals to benefit from a longer life.

The continuous improvements of our healthcare system will be the most important factor, together with what we eat and drink, for the increase of the expected lifetime to be beneficial for us.

Our politicians need to start building new pension fund systems adapted for the future of seriously longer life expectancy.

On the positive side, many of us will be able to work longer, and hence, maybe this will at least partly cover the increased cost of the equation for our societies.

My subject during my PhD studies and during my early working period was focused on radiation physics, with special reference to diagnostic imaging. I have worked with most of the imaging techniques and methods that exist today.

During my close to eight years as a hospital physicist at a large radiology department, I enjoyed being involved in the day-to-day clinical questions and challenges.

The focus for me and my small team at the time was to optimize image quality in order to increase the diagnostic accuracy for the radiologist to become as specific as possible in their diagnostic work.

The neuroradiologists at the department especially stimulated me and taught me about the brain and spine anatomy and its different functions. We were all eager to improve the image quality in order to continuously increase the diagnostic capabilities.

The fact that we had a skilled and very engaged neurosurgical department meant a lot for the continuous desire to stay at the forefront of diagnostic imaging.

After having finished my doctor's degree in medical science, I was seriously thinking of starting to study medicine to become a neuroradiologist. Family reasons stopped me from doing this, but my interest and curiosity in the medical discipline have never disappeared.

During my time as a hospital physicist and during the 25 years at GE HealthCare, I was heavily involved in both clinical as well as technical matters in the early days of mammography screening, computerized tomography (CT), magnetic resonance imaging (MRI), and positron-emission tomography (PET). With PET, there is also a need for automated radio chemistry development in order to make PET a more practical modality for use outside the leading university hospital sphere. It was very exciting and stimulating work and always in very close collaboration with clinical teams.

During my final 10 years at GE HealthCare, I had a role as EMEA (Europe, the Middle East, and Africa) research manager for our clinical collaborations with leading institutions around the world using all types of imaging and analysis tools that were within the scope of GE HealthCare.

In this role, I came in contact with a broad spectrum of scientists through the many research projects my team and I were involved in. These clinical collaborations led to a much broader research field for me and my team than just the imaging part. This meant a lot for my continuous interest and curiosity in biology, genetics, and the way different organs in our bodies function together.

When I look back, I think that it was during this time I started to build up an interest in the who, what, and when of medical developments throughout history, and the background of different medical and MedTech developments that has taken place during the last three to four decades.

What were and are the drivers in medical and MedTech developments, looking back into history, and what challenges and developments can we expect in the future?

Can we from the knowledge we have gained today, extrapolate into the future, and say something about the future of medicine and MedTech?

It is my ambition to try to shed some light on these questions with this book.

Being a radiation physicist by education, maybe you as a reader are wondering why a physicist is starting a project like this. Maybe a medical doctor would be a far better person to write this type of book.

I myself have had and still have the same thoughts and doubts.

Still, I think it is worth trying, as the subject is interesting, and medicine and healthcare are of interest to a broad audience, and for sure, it will expand my own knowledge from where I stand today.

What became the starting point for this book project?

I think it was when I decided to learn more about artificial intelligence (AI). This is close to three years ago.

After retiring from GE HealthCare, I started my own consultancy company and mainly focused on supporting new start-ups in order to help them go from the research level to the clinical and marketing level. Moreover, I have been and still am reviewing and evaluating research grant applications for Vinnova (the innovation authority in Sweden) and SSF (the Strategic Research Foundation in Sweden).

I started to feel that I needed more knowledge about AI, as this became a growing tool in several research projects that I evaluated.

I have been following the developments of AI within radiology, as a tool for qualification and quantification in readings from radiology images, but had ignored the use and development of AI in other disciplines, like drug development and, generally, bioscience.

I looked around for different courses and found a suitable lecture series at the Senior University in Stockholm. I signed up for this course but was very disappointed when the course was fully booked and I got a very high reserve place number that I did not have any hope of receiving a seat.

Instead, I looked at the season program for the fall of 2019 at the Senior University in Stockholm, but I did not find any course that excited me in the autumn/fall of 2019 program except the AI course I did not get a seat on.

What I did observe, though, was that the program did not include anything around developments in medicine and MedTech, which I thought would be of interest to an audience aged 55 years and upward.

Just by a spontaneous idea, I put together a suggestion for a lecture series on the developments within MedTech and its importance in medicine and sent this to the board of the Senior University in Stockholm.

Within a few days, I got a call from the board of the Senior University in Stockholm, and I hear a voice saying, "Bengt, you can start preparing yourself right away."

This call led to a course with six sessions and two hours at each gathering. To my surprise, 104 persons signed up, and there were never fewer than 102 students over 55 years during any of the lectures.

The lecture series was, of course, canceled during 2020 and 2021 due to the coronavirus pandemic, but it is likely that the lectures will be repeated in the fall of 2023.

Some of my students stimulated me to write a book with the lecture series as the basis. The suggestion led to the start of the project in early 2021.

I have always wondered how and when medicine moved forward or transferred from mysticism or religion to become a science. Moreover, when and how did technology become an integral part of medical development, and what were the driving mechanisms behind this development?

I was working as a hospital physicist during the early 1970s and into the late 1980s, and I took part in this journey as a researcher during the era when specialized X-ray techniques, like mammography, CT, the new MRI, PET, and single-photon emission computerized tomography (SPECT), were developed and clinically introduced. These techniques were, for sure, quantum leaps, as seen from a diagnostic point of view, and have had a profound impact on the patients.

During this time, diagnostic imaging also developed from being film-based to stepwise becoming fully digital.

I am convinced that the accelerated pace of today's developments will continue to renew and create new and improved methods for the benefit of people all over the world as well as in the future. The different techniques will also become miniaturized and the usage simplified in order to reach all areas of our planet.

Most likely, this will happen at an even faster pace than what we have seen until now.

The way I have looked at new developments is from the perspective of incremental steps and large steps that I call quantum leaps. Many of the incremental steps are maybe, at first sight, not so impressive, but they are essential in order to build new knowledge and build momentum for the coming bigger steps (quantum leaps).

As an example, the first CT scanner was a head-only scanner, but after a short time, it developed into a scanner for whole-body applications. The first CT dedicated to brain imaging, developed by Godfrey Hounsfield and Allan McLeod Cormack, was certainly a quantum leap, while the expansion toward whole-body application was more of an incremental step.

When I have been looking at different development steps through the history of medicine and MedTech developments, I have looked for quantum leap developments as well as incremental development steps, especially when I look at MedTech. Today's developments are often and increasingly coming from clinical and medical questions, and it is very common today that developments are done by multidisciplinary teams with a long list of different specialties in order to solve a specific medical problem or question.

Going back only 50 years, this was very rare, as we used to work much more in different silos before we eventually integrated these silos to form a clinical solution.

In this book, I will highlight the most important medical and MedTech steps that have been driving our developments toward our present knowledge and toward future major new developments.

I hope you will be stimulated to learn more and enjoy reading my attempt in this huge and exciting field.

Throughout time, scientists have spent immeasurable hours and resources hunting for medical advancements that will save the lives of sick people. When they encounter breakthroughs, like the ones of the 21st century, we can see how important their work is for every one of us. Scientific research is a rather slow process but a very important and necessary process for the safety

What We Should Really Worry About

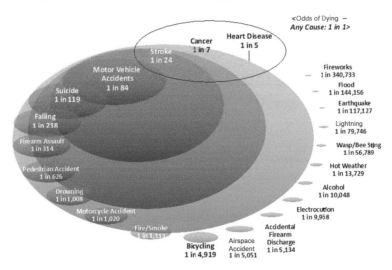

Figure 1   The things in life that are most dangerous in our lifetime and critical for our well-being are all connected to our health situation, as can be seen earlier, heart disease, cancer, and stroke. Data from the USA. (National Safety Council, 2003)[2]

of the patients being diagnosed and treated. Although some breakthroughs aren't immediately usable, the knowledge being built will most likely become relevant as scientists and researchers continue their work.[1, 2]

Treating and even curing diseases through scientific breakthroughs in order to improve the quality of life is on the rise. What a great time to be alive!

As you can see in Figure 1, the three highest risk factors for having a short life are due to diseases. The healthcare offered today reduces the three risk factors considerably compared to the data from 2003.

Let's start this story by looking both backward in history but also forward to see the mankind's progress when it comes to health and healthcare. Let's just keep in mind that not everyone around the world can enjoy this progress today. We have a lot more work to do before the world's population can benefit from the same privileges some of us can enjoy.

The main principel to follow is in my view what we call "*evidence based medicine*". **Welcome to an exciting journey together!**

Reference List, Preface

1 https://en.wikipedia.org/wiki/Medicine
2 National Safety Council 2003 data, printed in National Geographic.

AUTHOR

I was born in Malmö, in the south of Sweden, in 1949. I grew up as a single child with my mother but without my father. I know about him, but we never met in person. He did not want to have any contact with us. My mother was very caring, and I never lacked anything during my youth, and I had all the stimulation I could have wished for, thanks to my mother and my nanny and her family. During the 1950s in Sweden, life was easy, and my nanny took a lot of interest in my education. She stimulated and pushed me toward theoretical studies, while my own thoughts, and probably my mother's as well, were toward something more practical. I did not want to be different, and among my friends and in the vicinity where we lived, there was nobody who went to higher education.

My nanny, though, was a strong woman, and she won the educational discussion, and I ended up at the University in Lund.

I was also very lucky, as the late Olof Palme was the school minister those days, and he saw to it that people from the lower social classes in Sweden, which we belonged to, got the chance to enter higher education, with the possibility to get very favorable student loans. My mother was at first very nervous about these arrangements but gave in when I had all the loan agreements settled.

When I came to the University in Lund, I studied mathematics, physics, and finally, radiation physics. I took my basic university degree after three years of studies. These three years were probably some of the most important years in my youth.

The PhD studies started in Linköping, a young university those days. After one year, my research institute nominated me for a summer student position at the High Energy Physics Department at CERN in Geneva, Switzerland. Sweden can send three summer students to CERN every year. It was a privilege to be invited, and I got so inspired to be able to spend three and a half months in CERN outside Geneva. My boss at CERN wanted me to learn high-energy physics but also to enjoy and see everything in the beautiful Swiss countryside and mountains.

I learned new things every day, listened to very clever people daily, and made friends for life. It was for sure a very lucky time of my life.

So after one year as a PhD student, I found myself en route to becoming a high-energy physicist. A bit surprising, in fact, and something I never could have dreamt of.

When I was about to return to CERN a year later, I realized that there were not many places to live if you wanted to pursue a high-energy physicist career. Therefore, in spite of the first fantastic time at CERN a year before, I think this was why I started to lean toward medical physics. My PhD studies now moved forward with high speed until I got an offer to become a hospital physicist at the department of radiology in Linköping. It certainly slowed down my PhD studies, but I accepted the position.

I then started maybe the most important step in my career, the chance to work with the clinical radiology team. After some extra years, I finished the PhD and defended my thesis.

I was one of the physicists involved in the mammography screening program in Sweden, and this gave me an entry point for the MedTech industry.

After about five years as a hospital physicist, I accepted a position in the industry with GE HealthCare.

I had many different positions at GE HealthCare, like technical service manager and commercial positions, but the most interesting have been the ones leading the MRI modality in EMEA and the leadership for the research initiative, building collaborations with leading research sites in Europe and some other places in the world.

GE HealthCare sponsored our partners, and together, we went for research grants all over the world. The condition for the collaboration was that GE would lead and coordinate the collaborations. Accordingly, my team and I had a very tough job with endless amounts of travel. This job was the most challenging I ever had but also the most rewarding in the form of learning and lifetime friendships with many leading researchers within the field of healthcare.

In the summer of 2012, I left GE after 25 years. Today, I am retired but working approximately half time with different consulting jobs, lecturing, and writing a book.

I am very grateful and proud of all the fantastic opportunities I have been given throughout my life and have tried to fulfill my tasks with energy and dedication.

I have certainly been rewarded and have been able to enjoy life, work, and the family around me more than I could ever dream of. The next goal is, on top of finishing this book, to continue to engage in exciting projects and spend most of my time with my family.

Part 1

HEALTHCARE IN HISTORIC TIMES

1

PREHISTORIC MEDICINE AND ANCIENT MEDICINE HISTORY

1.1 The Big Bang, the Earth, the Evolutions, and the Revolutions

1.1.2 The Cognitive Revolution

About 14 billion years ago, our universe was created, and matter, energy, time, and space were erected in what we today call the Big Bang. These events are described by physicists. New advanced telescopes being sent out into space will maybe be able to see all the way back to the Big Bang, which most likely will give new insight into the Big Bang.

Approximately 300,000 years after matter and energy were created, they started to unite in complex structures called atoms. The atoms, in turn, built molecules. The description and research of these events led to the science of chemistry.

Approximately 4 billion years ago on a planet called Earth, specific molecules started to unite in complex structures called organisms. The story and research about organisms are called biology.

About 70,000 years ago, an organism called *Homo sapiens* started to build even more complex structures called cultures. These cultural developments are called history.

According to a new study from the University of Washington (United States), the Denisovans had a certain role in our evolutionary history; they cross-bred with our ancestors (*Homo sapiens*) at least twice. As a result, they left their imprint on our genome, which adds another twist to the already complex story of the dispersal of humans throughout Asia and the rest of the planet since they left Africa.

What this new work, led by the researcher Sharon Browning, from the Department of Bioinformatics at the University of Washington, notes is that Denisovans mixed with *Homo sapiens* in two different episodes in history.[1]

Three different and very important revolutions took place in our history.

- The Cognitive Revolution kick-started about 70,000 years ago. Three different humans lived side by side in the south of Africa during this time, and eventually, the *Homo sapiens* became the surviving family of the three types of humans. It is believed to be because they managed to remember things and draw conclusions from these memories long before this became part of the human DNA.[2, 3]

DOI: 10.1201/9781003393320-2

- The Agricultural Revolution started about 12,000 years ago. It is also called the Neolithic Revolution and is best described as the transformation of human societies from hunting and gathering to farming.[4, 5]
- The Scientific Revolution started 500 years ago and has been ongoing ever since. The Scientific Revolution was a series of events that marked the emergence of modern science during the early modern period when developments in mathematics, physics, astronomy, biology (including human anatomy), and chemistry transformed the views of society about nature.

People began using experiments and mathematics to understand mysteries. New discoveries were made, and old beliefs began to be proven wrong.

This revolution has had a huge impact on our lives as we now base our knowledge on verified research and not on perceptions, thoughts, or religious conventions.[6, 7]

1.2   The Medical History

1.2.1   The Prehistoric Period: 2.5 Million Years Ago to 1200 BC

There are many questions that come to one's mind when we think about the Prehistoric Period, focusing on human medicine and healthcare. The great difference in knowledge compared to our insights today are obvious, but what were the milestones, and why did these things occur and lead us to the systematic build of our knowledge that has occurred ever since? What were the reasons we moved away from the theories and beliefs that the god's anger or other mystical theories were the reasons for human body problems at this time?

Or is it the other way around, that due to our lack of knowledge and explanations, we believed in different religious theories?

My belief is that the very short life expectancy during the early days of mankind was a very strong driver for learning more about human health in order to live longer.

The evolution of the early *Homo sapiens* with the greater brains and phase 3 revolution that started approximately 500 years ago, called the Scientific Revolution, led to an accelerated development phase for medicine and healthcare.

As we will see, the road ahead was both bumpy and very long.

The Prehistoric Period, approximately 2.5 million years ago to 1200 BC, when there was human life but before records documented human activity, is generally categorized into three archaeological periods: Stone Age, Bronze Age, and Iron Age.

As there is scarce or no documentation from this period, our knowledge is based on artifacts, human remains, and to some extent, primitive people.

The first known writing system appeared approximately 5,300 years ago, and it took thousands of years for a writing system to be widely adopted.

Herb medicine is the earliest type of medicine. Proof via paintings has been found, for instance, in the cave of Lascaux in the south of France. These cave paintings are dated to be from approximately 15,000 years BC.

Diseases were, during the earliest times, believed to be caused by angry gods because of the way the people lived their lives. The impact of witchcraft and later religions on the way people lived were, consequently, of high impact.

One of the oldest known therapeutic methods in medicine is *trepanation.*

In ancient times, holes were drilled into a persons skull who was behaving in what was considered an abnormal way to let out what people believed were evil spirits.

Evidence of trepanation has been found in prehistoric human remains from the Neolithic Age (Stone Age, approximately 10,000 years BC) and times onward (see Figure 1.1).

While surgical practices, such as trepanations, are well attested since the first stages of the European Neolithic Age, the amputation of limbs in prehistoric periods has not been well- documented until the case presented here. The particularly well-preserved remains of an aged male were recently uncovered in the Neolithic site (4900–4700 BC) of Buthiers–Boulancourt in

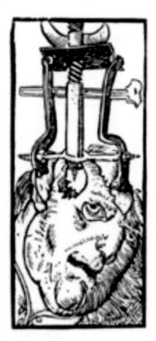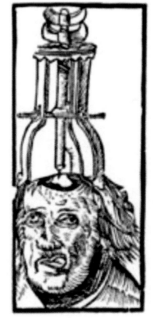

Figure 1.1   Trepanation. (commons.wikimedia.org)[8]

the vicinity of Paris, France. It was already noticed in situ that the distal part of the left humerus was abnormal, and this led us to the hypothesis of a partially healed surgical amputation. The further investigations reported here confirm a traumatic origin and partial healing of scar tissue after surgery. This suggested that the patient survived. It also proves the remarkable medical skills developed during prehistoric times. If indeed this man benefited from some form of community care, this would indicate the level of social solidarity in Western Europe almost 7,000 years ago.

Evidence also suggests that trepanation was primitive emergency surgery after head wounds to remove shattered bits of bone from a fractured skull and clean out the blood that often pools under the skull after a blow to the head. Hunting accidents, falls, wild animals, and weapons, such as clubs or spears, could have caused such injuries. Trepanations appear to have been most common in areas where weapons that could produce skull fractures were used.

The primary theories for the practice of trepanation in ancient times include spiritual purposes, like driving out demons and releasing evil spirits. Trepanning was also used as a treatment for epilepsy, headaches, head wounds, and mental disorders.

Exorcism: Tribal doctors and witch doctors would try to drive out the evil spirits that made people sick.

Skeletal evidence has been found demonstrating trepanation.

Life expectancy during this era was only approximately 20 years.[9]

1.3   Egypt: 4000–1600 BC

Temples were places of worship, medical schools, and hospitals.

Only the priests could read the medical knowledge from the god Thoth. Magicians were also healers, and there was a belief that demons caused diseases.

The medical prescriptions were written on papyrus. The Egyptians had rather advanced knowledge of anatomy.

Strong antiseptics were used to prevent the decay of health conditions.

Gauze, like today's surgical gauze, found on mummies indicated some modern use similar to today's use. Proof of diseases, like arthritis, kidney stones, and arteriosclerosis, have been found.

Some medical practices used in ancient Egypt are still used today: enemas, circumcision preceding marriage (4000 BC), splinted fractures, and bloodletting.

Egyptian Eye of Horus: The magic eye is an Egyptian myth (approximately 5,000 years ago).

In one myth, when Set and Horus were fighting for the throne after Osiris's death, Set gouged out Horus's left eye. Most of the eye was restored by either Hathor or Thoth. When Horus's eye was recovered, he offered it to his father, Osiris, in hopes of restoring his life. Hence, the Eye of Horus was often used to symbolize sacrifice, healing, restoration, and protection.

The Eye of Horus is today used on amulets as a symbol of protection against diseases and evils.[10]

In the very early civilizations, like the one in Egypt, 3000 BC, a rather sophisticated type of medicine was developed. It was well organized in disciplines like surgery, dentistry, anatomy, and pharmacology. The knowledge was partly based on empirical experience that common medical diseases and conditions were due to supernatural powers.

The universal genius and polymath Imhotep has been said to be the world's first medical doctor. Additionally, he was an architect, astronomer, and an engineer. Imhotep is also said to be the designer of the first pyramid in Egypt, the stepstone pyramid in Saqqara, rather close to Giza. This first pyramid was built to honor Pharaoh Djoser.

The Edwin Smith Papyrus is an ancient Egyptian medical text named after the dealer who bought it in 1862 and the oldest known surgical treatise on trauma. This document may have been a manual of military surgery and describes 48 cases of injuries, fractures, wounds, dislocations, and tumors. It dates to dynasties 16–17 of the Second Intermediate Period in ancient Egypt, approximately 1600 BC.

For instance, the Edwin Smith Papyrus describes how to close wounds with sutures, how to stop bleedings with raw meat, and how to cure infections with honey.

The Edwin Smith Papyrus is unique among the four principal medical papyri in existence that survive today. While other papyri, such as the Ebers Papyrus and London Medical Papyrus, are medical texts, the Edwin Smith Papyrus presents a rational and scientific approach to medicine in ancient Egypt, in which medicine and magic do not conflict. Magic would be more prevalent had the cases of illnesses been mysterious, such as internal disease. Sometimes, it is said that the Edwin Smith Papyrus was written by Imhotep, but no real proof for this has been found.

In the Ebers Papyrus, the neurological disease dementia was mentioned for the first time. It took all the way to 1797 before the French psychiatrist Philippe Pinel, who was called the father of modern psychiatry, used the word *dementia* as a description of a person with an intellectual deficit, literally, a person who was "out of his mind," in Latin.[11–13]

Personal Anecdote

Many years ago, during my university study times, I traveled frequently to Egypt, as archeology was a big interest of mine those days.

My friend and I traveled together with a guide on a camel from Giza, outside Cairo, to Saqqara to the staircase pyramid with the tomb of

Pharaoh Djoser. It was a tough ride due to the heat and the not-always-comfortable camelback that we were not used to. Arriving at Saqqara, we found shade at the entrance to the tomb.

To our surprise, there was a salesman in front of a wooden box with a water bath in which many different drink bottles were swimming. Cooled drinks in the middle of a dessert! Was it a mirage, or had we already arrived in paradise?

One drink that we could not find in the box was Coca-Cola. According to the salesman, he had an equivalent drink called Pepsi cola. We had never heard of it then, but we tested it, and ever since, I have always chosen Pepsi instead of Coca-Cola, not because of the taste or advertising but due to the fantastic memory from Saqqara.

A Pepsi cola at the foot of the stepstone pyramid in Saqqara is unbeatable, at least for me.

Sir William Osler (Canadian doctor, 1849–1919) described Imhotep as "the first figure of a physician to stand out clearly from the mists of antiquity." His medical practices deviated from the use of magic and prayer that other Egyptian healers used and were remarkably advanced for the time.

The reason that we know so many details from ancient Egypt is the discovery and deciphering of the Rosetta Stone in 1822.

At the British Museum in London, the remarkable stone called the Rosetta Stone has its home today.

When it was discovered, nobody knew how to read ancient Egyptian hieroglyphs. Because the inscriptions say the same thing in three different scripts, and scholars could still read ancient Greek, the Rosetta Stone became a valuable key to deciphering the hieroglyphs. The importance of this to Egyptology is amazing.

The very difficult work of deciphering hieroglyphs from the Rosetta Stone was done by Thomas Young (1773–1829), a British polymath who also made notable contributions to the fields of vision, light, solid mechanics, energy, physiology, language, musical harmony, and Egyptology.

The reason that the work was very difficult was that the Rosetta Stone was found rather incomplete, and hence, the text in three different languages was incomplete.[14]

The Hearst Papyrus, also called the Hearst Medical Papyrus, is one of the medical papyri of ancient Egypt. It was named after Phoebe Hearst. The papyrus contains 18 pages of medical prescriptions written in hieratic Egyptian writing, concentrating on treatments for problems dealing with the urinary system, blood, hair, and bites. It is dated to the first half of the 2nd millennium BC. It is considered an important manuscript, but some doubts persist about its authenticity.[15]

Note: The historian Herodotus, born in 484 BC in Minor Asia, which is Turkey today, is a very important source of information.

Herodotus called the Egyptians "the healthiest people in the World." The reasons for this were their advanced health system and their dry and very stable climate.

Ancient Egypt still had several diseases, despite the stable climate, and this was the beginning of a health system:

- Many people worked by the Nile, where the risk was high for getting deadly parasites or becoming sick with malaria.
- From grave findings, it has been discovered that many people suffered from malnutrition in spite of the fact that agriculture produced food in excess.
- Child mortality was high, and only one-third of the population reached adulthood.
- The life expectancy was low: 35 years for men and 30 years for women.

1.4   India: 700–600 BC

Ayurveda, also known as the Indian system of medicine, is an alternative medicine system with historical roots in the Indian subcontinent.

The theory and practice of Ayurveda is pseudoscientific.

The main classical Ayurveda texts begin with accounts of the transmission of medical knowledge from the gods to sages and then to human physicians. Sushruta Samhita wrote his *Sushruta's Compendium,* a text on medicine and surgery, and one of the most important treatises on this subject to survive in the ancient world. He is known today as the father of Indian medicine and the father of plastic surgery for inventing and developing surgical procedures. Therapies are typically based on complex herbal compounds, minerals, and metal substances perhaps under the influence of early Indian alchemy or *rasa shastra,* which details processes by which various metals, mineral sand, and other substances, including mercury, are purified and combined with herbs in an attempt to treat illnesses.

Ancient Ayurveda texts also taught surgical techniques, including rhinoplasty, kidney stone extraction, sutures, and the extraction of foreign objects. Ayurveda has been adapted for Western consumption, notably by Baba Hari Dass in the 1970s and Maharishi Ayurveda in the 1980s.

Some scholars teach us that Ayurveda originated in prehistoric times and that some of the concepts of Ayurveda have existed from the time of the Indus Valley Civilization (3300–1300 BC) or a bit earlier.

Ayurveda developed significantly during the Vedic Period, 1500–500 BC, and later, some of the non-Vedic systems, such as Buddhism and Jainism, also developed medical concepts and practices that appear in the classical

Ayurveda texts. *Dosha* is one of the three substances that are believed to be present in a person's body.

The *dosha* balance is emphasized, and suppressing natural urges is considered unhealthy and claimed to lead to illness. Ayurveda treatises describe three elemental substances, *vata, pitta,* and *kapha,* and state that balance of the *doshas* results in health, while imbalance results in disease. Ayurveda treatises divide medicine into eight canonical components. Ayurveda practitioners had developed various medicinal preparations and surgical procedures from at least the beginning of the Common Era. To me, the *dosha* theory and its substances sound like the humorism theory, where the balance in the chemical systems regulating human behavior impacts our well-being. Humorism is to be discussed later in the book.

There is no good evidence that Ayurveda is effective in treating any disease. Ayurvedic preparations have been found to contain lead, mercury, and arsenic, substances known to be harmful to humans. In a 2008 study, close to 21% of US- and Indian-manufactured patent Ayurvedic medicines sold through the internet were found to contain toxic levels of heavy metals, specifically lead, mercury, and arsenic. The public health implications of such metallic contaminants in India are unknown.

According to modern Ayurveda sources, the origin of the Ayurveda health program/medicine goes back to approximately 5000 BC. Reconstructive surgery was done in India around 800 BC.

> *Note 1:* The Indian Medical Association (IMA) characterizes the practice of modern medicine by Ayurvedic practitioners as quackery/health fraud.[16]
>
> *Note 2:* In a recent article in *Medical News Today,* Ayurvedic medicine is an alternative or complementary form of medicine, which may be useful in treating various conditions, such as GERD (frequent heartburn), diabetes, erectile dysfunction, and more.

Ayurvedic practitioners have been using plants, diet, exercise, and lifestyle to treat various conditions for more than 3,000 years, and they consider it a holistic, whole-body healing system.

Research into the effectiveness of Ayurvedic medicine is ongoing, and professionals need further clinical evidence to support its use in treating many conditions.[17]

1.5   Traditional Chinese Medicine: 900 BC–AD 1800

Traditional Chinese medicine (TCM) has been described as fraught with pseudoscience, with most of its treatments having no logical mechanism of action.

TCM is said to be based on the *Compendium of Materia Medica* and *Huangdi Neijing.* Several Chinese authors have written texts on the treatment of many diseases in a question and answer form. The original text covers the theoretical foundation of Chinese Medicine and its diagnostic and treatment methods. *Huangdi Neijing*, the "Yellow Emperor" was one of the earliest original medical texts in China.

The practice includes various forms of herbal medicine, acupuncture, cupping therapy, *gua* massage, bonesetter exercise (*gigong*), and dietary therapy.

TCM is widely used in the East Asian cultural sphere, where it has a long history. Subsequently, it is now also practiced outside of China. One of the basic principles of TCM is that the body's vital energy is circulating through channels called meridians, having branches connected to bodily organs and functions. The concept of vital energy is pseudoscientific. Concepts of the body and of disease used in TCM reflect its ancient origins and its emphasis on dynamic processes over material structure, like the humoral theory of ancient Greece and ancient Rome.

China also developed a large body of traditional medicine. Much of the philosophy of traditional Chinese medicine is derived from empirical observations of disease. According to Taoist physicians, illness reflects the classical Chinese belief that individual human experiences express the reason to disease. These causative principles, whether material, essential, or mystical, correlate as the expression of the natural order of the universe.

The foundational text about Chinese medicine is the *Huangdi Neijing* or *Yellow Emperor's Inner Canon*, written in the 5th century to the 3rd century BCE. Before the Common Era (BCE) is the year notation for the Gregorian calendar. Near the end of the 2nd century CE, Zhang Zhonging, a Chinese pharmacologist, physician, inventor, and writer of the Eastern Han dynasty, wrote a treatise on cold damage, which contains the earliest known reference to the *Neijing Suwen*, also known as *Basic Questions*, covering the theoretical foundation of Chinese medicine and its diagnostic methods. Zhang Zhonging lived from AD 150 to AD 219.

The Jin dynasty practitioner and advocate of acupuncture Huangfu (AD 215–282) also quotes the *Yellow Emperor* in his *Jiayijing*, year 265. During the Tang dynasty, the *Suwen* was expanded and revised and is now the best representation of the foundational roots of traditional Chinese medicine. Traditional Chinese medicine, which is based on the use of herbal medicine, acupuncture, massage, and other forms of therapy, has been practiced in China for thousands of years.

In the 18th century, during the Qing dynasty, there was a proliferation of popular books as well as more advanced encyclopedias on traditional medicine. Jesuit missionaries introduced Western science and medicine to the royal court, although the Chinese physicians ignored them.[18]

Finally, in the 19th century, Western medicine was introduced at the local level by Christian medical missionaries from the London Missionary

Society (in Britain), the Methodist Church (in Britain), and the Presbyterian Church (in the United States). Benjamin Hobson (1816–1873), in 1839, set up a highly successful Wai Ai Clinic in Guangzhou, China. The Hong Kong College of Medicine for Chinese was founded in 1887 by the London Missionary Society, with its first graduate in 1892 being Sun Yat-sen, who later led the Chinese Revolution (1911). The Hong Kong College of Medicine for Chinese was the forerunner of the School of Medicine of the University of Medicine, which started in 1911.

Because of the social custom that men and women should not be near one another, the women of China were reluctant to be treated by male doctors. The missionaries sent women doctors, such as Dr. Mary Hannah Fulton (1854–1927). Supported by the Foreign Missions Board of the Presbyterian Church (United States), she, in 1902, founded the first medical college for women in China, the Hackett Medical College for Women, in Guangzhou.

When reading the Chinese classics, it is important for scholars to examine these works from the Chinese perspective. Historians have noted two key aspects of Chinese medical history: understanding conceptual differences when translating the term *shén* and observing history from the perspective of cosmology rather than biology.

In Chinese classical texts, the term *shén* is the closest historical translation to the English word *body* because it sometimes refers to the physical human body in terms of being weighed or measured, but the term is to be understood as an "ensemble of functions" encompassing both the human psyche and emotions. This concept of the human body is opposed to the European duality of a separate mind and body. It is critical for scholars to understand the fundamental differences in concepts of the body in order to connect the medical theory of the classics to the "human organism" it is explaining.[19]

Chinese scholars established a correlation between the cosmos and the human organism. The basic components of cosmology, qi, yin yang (Figure 1.2), and the Five Phase theory, were used to explain health and disease in texts such as *Huangdi Nejling* is one of the original medical texts from China. Yin and Yang are the changing factors in cosmology, with qi as the vital force or energy of life. The Five Phase theory, *Wu Xing*, of the Han dynasty, contains the elements wood, fire, earth, metal, and water. By understanding medicine from a cosmology perspective, historians can better understand Chinese medical and social classifications, such as gender, which was defined by domination or remission of yang in terms of yin.

These two distinctions are imperative when analyzing the history of traditional Chinese medical science.

A majority of Chinese medical history written after the classical canons comes in the form of primary source case studies where academic physicians record the illness of a particular person and the healing techniques used as

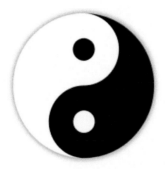

Figure 1.2 Yin and yang is a Chinese philosophical concept that describes opposite but interconnected forces. (wikipedia.org, *Huangdi Nejling*, Yin and Yang)[20]

well as their effectiveness. Historians have noted that Chinese scholars wrote these studies instead of "books of prescriptions or advice manuals;" in their historical and environmental understanding, no two illnesses were alike, so the healing strategies of the practitioner were unique every time to the specific diagnosis of the patient. Medical case studies existed throughout Chinese history, but "individually authored and published case history" was a prominent creation of the Ming dynasty. An example of such case studies would be the literati physician Cheng Congzhou's collection of 93 cases published in 1644:

- The Chinese monitored the pulse rate to determine the condition of the body.
- They cured the whole body by curing the spirit and nourishing it.
- They have the first recorded pharmacy of herbs.
- They used acupuncture and acupressure.
- They began searching for organic causes of disease.
- The average life span is 20 to 30 years.
- Acupuncture.
- They treated diseases with stone tools.

1.5.1 Summary and Thoughts around Chinese Ancient Medicine, 1700 BC–AD 220

1. Religion prohibited the dissection of the body of the ancient Chinese.
2. The Chinese believed that you had to treat both the body and spirit: yin and yang.
3. They discovered a pharmacopeia of medications based on herbs.
4. Therapies included acupuncture.
5. Holistic medicine stresses treating the entire patient, mind, body, and soul.[21]

1.6   Babylon: 1800–600 BC

Ancient Babylonian medicine made use of a great number of materials—primarily plant life and animal products (sometimes, feces), along with minerals. Many of the materials used in these prescriptions remain unidentified. These ingredients could be administered in several forms, including salves, rubbing oils, drinks, pills, wraps, and enemas. No evidence indicates the use of any of these materials in anesthetics, however (which, as a side note, would mean any patient undergoing surgery would have to endure high levels of pain). In addition, while mental disorders were primarily treated with magic, physicians also made use of herbal remedies.

Some texts detail prescriptions for a salve to help sun disease, which was likely sunburn. One document details treating kidney problems by inserting a bronze tube in the urethra and blowing drugs through.

The following is another prescription for kidney disease from a Babylonian medical text (the unknown materials are anglicized and left untranslated):

> Crush together imhur-lim, myrrh, ostrich eggshell, black frit—for 3 days in fish brine, for 3 days in drawn wine, and for 3 days in pomegranate juice—he keeps drinking it and he will improve.

The following is a prescription intended to treat intestinal bloating and flatulence:

> Heat in premium beer nlnu, mountain plant, hasu, nuhurtu, juniper, kukru, sumlalu, ballukku, cuttings of aromatics, field-clod, plants—filter and cool them, add oil into the mixture—pour it into his anus and he will recover.

1.6.1   Magic and Spiritualism

Magic played a central role in ancient Babylonian medicine, with both the exorcist and the physician utilizing the supernatural to a large degree. Even natural medical treatment would typically be administered alongside some sort of spell or incantation. For example, the following is an incantation warning debris to leave the eye before the physician intervenes to remove it himself:

> Eyes with the porous blood vessel, why have you been blurred by chaff, thorns, sursurru-irait, or river algae? Rain down here like a star, keep falling here like a meteor, before the knife and scalpel of Gula reach you. An irreversible incantation, the incantation of Asalluhi-Marduk and the incantation of Ningirimma, master of spells, and Gula, master of healing arts, has cast it and I have taken it up.

Note the references to Gula, the goddess of healing. She is often referred to in magical incantations used in the spiritual aspects of ancient Babylonian medicine. However, these spells are more than just appeals to gods and spirits. They were a form of prose (unstructured poetry), often using symbolic language and repeating motifs. For example, in the incantation earlier, the exorcist calls for the debris (or perhaps tears) to rain down like a (shooting) star. Other common elements used by writers include repetition and short stories, as seen in the following incantation regarding a sore in the eye:

> The wind was blowing in heaven and a sore settled in a man's eye.
> It blew in from the distant heavens and a sore settled in a man's eye.
> A sore was found in the sick eyes. The eyes of that man are troubled—his eyes are blurred, and when by himself, that man cries bitterly.
> Nanmu noticed that man's illness:
> "Take crushed kasu, recite the Eridu incantation, bind the eye of that man."
> When Nammu touches the man's eye with her pure hand, may the wind which is swept into a man's eye be removed from his eye.

Standardization: The Babylonian healthcare system seems to have been rather well standardized, with some level of legal code.

The *Hammurabi Code* (c. 2000 BC), inscribed on an eight-foot-tall block of black diorite, covers doctor payment and malpractice. Lines 218 to 221, listed as follows, detail punishment for malpractice as well as proper payment for physicians:

- If the doctor has treated a man for a severe wound with lances of bronze and has caused the man to die, or has opened an abscess of the eye for a man and has caused the loss of the man's eye, one shall cut off his hands.
- If a doctor has treated the severe wound of a slave of a poor man with a bronze lances and has caused his death, he shall render slave for slave.
- If he has opened his abscess with a bronze lance and has made him lose his eye, he shall pay money, half his price.
- If a doctor has cured the shattered limb of a gentleman, or has cured the diseased bowel, the patient shall give five shekels of silver to the doctor.

These lines and others inscribed on the block indicate a widespread and rather standardized system of healthcare throughout ancient Babylonia.[22, 23]

The oldest Babylonian texts on medicine date back to the Old Babylonian Period in the first half of the 2nd millennium BC, years 2000 to 1000. The most extensive Babylonian medical text, however, is the *Diagnostic Handbook* written by the Ummânū, chief scholar, Esagil-kin-apli of Borsippa, during the reign of the Babylonian king Adad-apla-iddina (1069–1046 BC).

Along with contemporary Egyptian medicine, the Babylonians introduced the concepts of diagnosis, prognosis, physical examination, enemas, and prescription. In addition, the *Diagnostic Handbook* introduced the methods of therapy and etiology (cause or origin of a disease) and the use of empiricism, logic, and rationality in diagnosis, prognosis, and therapy. The text contains a list of medical symptoms and often detailed empirical observations, along with logical rules used in combining observed symptoms on the body of a patient with its diagnosis and prognosis.

The symptoms and diseases of a patient were treated through therapeutic means, such as bandages, creams, and pills. If a patient could not be cured physically, the Babylonian physicians often relied on exorcism to cleanse the patient from any curses. *Diagnostic Handbook* (Esagil-kin-apli's) was based on a logical set of axioms and assumptions, including the modern view that through the examination and inspection of the symptoms of a patient, it is possible to determine the patient's disease, its etiology, its future development, and the chances of the patient's recovery.

Esagil-kin-apli discovered a variety of illnesses and diseases and described their symptoms in his *Diagnostic Handbook*. These include the symptoms for many varieties of epilepsy and related ailments, along with their diagnosis and prognosis.[24]

1.7   Summary and Thoughts on the Prehistoric Era

1. Despite the beliefs that the knowledge from this part of human history and, specifically, the medicine/medical knowledge from the Prehistoric Period is rather limited, a few conclusions can be made.
2. The beliefs were that illnesses and diseases were a punishment from the gods. First physicians were witch doctors who treated illness with ceremonies.
3. During prehistoric times, herbs and plants were used as medicine. Foxglove plants (*Digitalis*) leaves were chewed to strengthen and slow the heart.
4. The knowledge about the human body, both anatomically and functionally, was very limited. The average life length was limited to around 30–35 years. In most parts of the world, it was not possible to talk about any healthcare at all.
5. Diseases were mainly seen as a punishment from angry gods following the lifestyle of the people. Mysticism and the influence of religion were dominating the whole prehistoric era.
6. The Babylonian healthcare system was organized rather well around several nice principles, like standardization of the healthcare system, accountability for the practicing doctors in case of malpractice, hygiene was strict, and so on. Still, it is clear from history that several treatments practiced were based on magic, mysticism, and spiritualism.

7. The Egyptian era was the first time when we can talk about a systematic approach to medicine as well as an organizational population-based healthcare system. Although it did not really reach the main population, it was still an important step toward what we today would call healthcare.

8. Egyptians were the first to keep accurate health records written on papyrus. Physicians were priests. Temples were used as places of worship, medical schools, and hospitals.

9. The possibilities for curing people from different diseases were, in general, very limited. The treatments were mainly focused on reducing pain and palliative directions. Mainly, extracts from plants and herbs were used, and their effect on serious diseases can be challenged or even questioned.

10. Medicine was rooted in religious or spiritual beliefs. Herbs and plants used as medicines were *Digitalis*, quinine, belladonna, atropine, and morphine.

11. There were documented ideas, such as washing and shaving a body before surgery. They used medicines to heal disease and learned the art of splinting fractures.

12. Primitive surgeries were used, but as the anatomy was not really known in detail, the results and benefits can be questioned. It is doubtful that anybody survived the trepanning surgery method. Such information is, unfortunately, not documented.

13. Remember that it would take merely 2,500 years before we were starting to build the needed knowledge, tools, and techniques in order to really make an impact on ordinary people and really be able to talk about a worldwide healthcare system.[25-26]

Let's continue to dig into the history of medicine and move on to modern medicine.

Reference List, Chapter 1

1 Yuval Noah Harari: *Sapiens. A Brief History of Mankind.* Natur & Kultur, 2014. In Swedish.
2 https://en.wikipedia.org/wiki/Cognitive_Revolution
3 Yuval Noah Harari: *Sapiens. A Brief History of Mankind.* Natur & Kultur, 2014. In Swedish.
4 https://en.wikipedia.org/wiki/Neolithic_Revolution
5 Yuval Noah Harari: *Sapiens. A Brief History of Mankind.* Natur & Kultur, 2014. In Swedish.
6 https://en.wikipedia.org/wiki/Scientific_Revolution
7 https://commons.wikimedia.org/wiki/Category:Trepanation
8 https://en.wikipedia.org/wiki/Edwin_Smith_Papyrus
9 https://en.wikipedia.org/wiki/Eye_of_Horus
10 https://en.wikipedia.org/wiki/Edwin_Smith_Papyrus

11 https://en.wikipedia.org/wiki/London_Medical_Papyrus
12 https://en.wikipedia.org/wiki/Ebers Papyrus
13 https://en.wikipedia.org/wiki/Thomas Young (scientist)
14 https://en.wikipedia.org/wiki/Hearst_papyrus
15 https://en.wikipedia.org/wiki/Ayurveda
16 Medically reviewed by Monisha Bhanote MD, FCAP, ABOIM, CCMS, YMTS. Written by Caitlin Geng on March 29, 2002.
17 https://en.wikipedia.org/wiki/Huangdi_Neijing
18 https://en.wikipedia.org/wiki/Shen_(Chinese_religion)
19 https://en.wikipedia.org/wiki/Yin_and_yang
20 https://patient.practicalpainmanagement.com/treatments/alternative/6-traditional-chinese-medicine-techniques
21 www.slideshare.net/Rivindu Wickramanayake/ babylonian-history-of-medicine-rivin
22 www.worldhistory.org/Gula/
23 https://en.wikipedia.org/wiki/Mesopotamia#Medicine
24 Prehistory, Wikipedia, the Free Encyclopedia.
25 www.worldhistory.org/Egyptian_Medicine/
26 https://bmcr.brynmawr.edu/2011/2011.08.37/

2

ANCIENT MEDICINE (700 BC–AD 476)

The history of medicine shows how societies have changed in their approach to illness and disease from ancient times to the present. Early medical traditions include those of Babylon, China, Egypt, and India. Sushruta, from India, introduced the concepts of medical diagnosis, the process of determining which disease or condition explains a person's symptoms and signs, and prognosis, a medical term for predicting the likely or expected development of a disease.[28, 29]

The Hippocratic Oath was written in ancient Greece in 500 BC and is a direct inspiration for oaths of office that physicians swear upon entry into the profession even today. In the Middle Ages, surgical practices inherited from the ancient masters were improved and then systematized in Rogerius's book *The Practice of Surgery*. Rogerius's work is brief and well-organized. It is also very practical and does not contain long citations from other medical authorities. Universities began systematic training of physicians around AD 1220 in Italy.[1]

The Hippocratic Oath is an oath of ethics historically taken by physicians. It is one of the most widely known Greek medical texts. In its original form, it requires a new physician to swear to several spiritual gods to uphold specific ethical standards. The oath is the earliest expression of medical ethics in the Western world, establishing several principles of medical ethics that remain of paramount significance today. These include the principles of medical confidentially and non-maleficence. As the seminal articulation of certain principles that continue to guide and inform medical practice, the ancient text is of more than historic and symbolic value. Swearing to a modified form of the oath remains a rite of passage for medical graduates in many countries and is a requirement enshrined in legal statutes of various jurisdictions, such that violations of the oath may carry criminal or other liability beyond the oath's symbolic nature.

The original oath was written in Ionic Greek, between the fifth and third centuries BC. Although it is traditionally attributed to the Greek doctor Hippocrates and is usually included in the *Hippocratic Corpus*, most modern scholars do not regard it as having been written by Hippocrates himself. The Greeks were the first to provide medical care for soldiers during battle. Early hospitals were usually placed in the homes of doctors. They were the first to create a public health part of government and develop sanitation systems.

DOI: 10.1201/9781003393320-3

Hippocrates and other doctors worked on the assumption that all diseases had a natural cause rather than a supernatural one. Priests believed that an illness, such as epilepsy, was caused by the gods.

Hippocrates believed that, with all other illnesses, it had a natural cause. The Hippocratic Oath is one of the oldest binding documents in history and gives a newly graduated doctor the opportunity to swear to uphold a set of professional ethical standards. It is the earliest expression of medical ethics in the Western world and established several principals of medical ethics that remain of paramount significance today. The document is generally attributed to Hippocrates, also known as Hippocrates II, although some argue that it may have been written after his death.

Here is a short and modernized version of the Hippocratic Oath

- I swear by Apollo Healer, by Asclepius, by Hygeia, by Panacea, and by all the gods and goddesses, making them my witnesses, that I will carry out, according to my ability and judgment, this oath, and this indenture.
- To hold my teacher in this art equal to my own parents; to make him partner in my livelihood; when he needs money to share mine with him; to consider his family as my own brothers, and to teach them this art, if they want to learn it, without fee or indenture; to impart precept, oral instruction, and all other instruction to my own sons, the sons of my teacher, and to indentured pupils who have taken the Healer's oath, but to nobody else.
- I will use those dietary regimens which will benefit my patients according to my greatest ability and judgment, and I will do no harm or injustice to them. Neither will I administer a poison to anybody when asked to do so, nor will I suggest such a course. Similarly, I will not give to a woman a pessary to cause abortion. But I will keep pure and holy both my life and my art. I will not use the knife, not even, verily, on sufferers from stone, but I will give place to such as are craftsmen therein.
- Into whatsoever houses I enter, I will enter to help the sick, and I will abstain from all intentional wrong-doing and harm, especially from abusing the bodies of man or woman, bond or free. And whatsoever I shall see or hear during, my profession, as well as outside my profession in my intercourse with men, if it be what should not be published abroad, I will never divulge, holding such things to be holy secrets.
- Now if I carry out this oath, and break it not, may I gain for ever reputation among all men for my life and for my art; but if I break it and forswear myself, may the opposite befall me.

Translation by W.H.S. Jones[1]

Aristotle (384–322 BC) started comparative anatomy.

Aristotle, known to be one of the greatest minds that ever existed, is indeed the godfather of evidence-based medicine.

Evidence-based medicine deemphasizes intuition, unsystematic clinical experience, and pathophysiologic rationale as sufficient grounds for clinical decision-making and stresses the examination of evidence from clinical research.

Aristotle's teachings of logic and philosophy have been a driving force that is continuously guiding medicine away from superstition and toward the scientific method.

Aristotle is principally known as a theoretical philosopher and logician, but he was also an excellent natural scientist.

In particular, he should probably be considered the first anatomist in the modern sense of this term and the originator of anatomy as a special branch of knowledge. Although it seems certain that he did not perform dissections of human adult cadavers, he examined human fetal material and, above all, made systematic analyses of animal bodies. His contribution to comparative anatomy, as well as to human anatomy, was essential.

Greeks believed that evil spirits or angry gods caused diseases and that the gods, such as Asclepius, son of Apollo, could heal and cure diseases. Sacrifice and prayer, often at Asclepius's shrine, were common methods of seeking a remedy.

Herbs and plants were used for healing. No other cure was available during this time.

The ancient Greeks were thirsty for logic and logic-based discussions, and they were curious about why things existed and why events happened. This curiosity paved the way for important developments in math and science. Ancient records show that they set up an early medical school in Cnidus in 700 BC. Here, they began the practice of observing patients who were sick. The Greeks were eager to study the causes of disease.[2]

Alkmaion lived around 500 BC and worked at the school in Cnidus. He wrote widely on medicine, although he was probably a philosopher of science rather than a doctor.

Without special examination, the brain offers no clue that it is the organ of the mind. Alkmaion was the first ancient scholar who recognized the human brain as the most important organ in the human body, connected with sensory organs; it was possible because he primarily recognized the construction of the optic nerve. Therefore, this philosopher initiated the approach to medicine called encephalometry.

Alkmaion regarded the brain as a place of intelligent mind, which in antiquity was not a frequent view. Alkmaion suggested the brain was the seat of understanding. Alkmaion could be called the father of neuroscience.[3, 4]

2.1 Humorism

The concept of humors (i.e., chemical systems regulating human behavior) became more prominent from the writing of medical theorist Alkmaion of Croton (c. 540–500 BC). His list of humorism was longer than just five liquids and included fundamental elements described by Empedocles, such as water, air, and earth. Some authors suggest that the concept of humorism may have origins in ancient Egyptian medicine or Mesopotamia, though it was not systemized until ancient Greek thinkers. The word *humor* is a translation of Greek χυμός or *chymos* (literally, "juice" or metaphorically, "flavor").[5]

Ancient Indian Ayurveda medicine had developed a theory of three so-called *doshas*, which they linked with the five elements: earth, water, fire, air, and ether. Hippocrates is the one usually credited with applying this idea to medicine. In contrast to Alkmaion, Hippocrates suggested that humors are vital bodily fluids, such as blood, yellow bile, phlegm, and black bile (he probably referred to blood composites in patients with bleeding internal organs). Alkmaion and Hippocrates postulated that an extreme excess or deficiency of any of the four humor bodily fluids in a person can be a sign of illness. Hippocrates and then Galen suggested that a moderate imbalance in the mixture of these fluids produces temperament (behavior) types. One of the treatises attributed to Hippocrates *On the Nature of Man* describes the theory as follows:

> The Human body contains blood, phlegm, yellow bile, and black bile. These are the things that make up its constitution and cause its pains and health. Health is primarily that state in which these constituent substances are in the correct proportion to each other, both in strength and quantity, and are well mixed. Pain occurs when one of the substances presents either a deficiency or an excess, or is separated in the body and not mixed with others.

2.1.1   The Four Humors

Even though the humorism theory had several models that used two, three, and five components, the most famous model consists of the four humors described by Hippocrates and then developed further by Galen. The four humors of Hippocratic medicine are black bile, yellow bile, phlegm, and blood. Each corresponds to one of the traditional four temperaments.

Based on Hippocratic medicine, it was believed that the four humors were to be in balanced proportions regarding the amount and strength of each humor for a body to be healthy. The proper blending and balance of the four humors were known as *eukrasia*. Imbalance and separation of humors lead to diseases.

> *Blood*: The blood was believed to be produced exclusively by the liver. It was associated with a sanguine nature (enthusiastic, active, and social).

Yellow bile. Excess yellow bile was thought to produce aggression, and consequently, excess anger causes liver derangement and imbalances in the humors.

Black bile. The word *melancholy* derives from Greek, meaning "black bile." Depression was attributed to excess or unnatural black bile secreted by the spleen. Cancer was also attributed to an excess of black bile concentrated in a specific area.

Phlegm. Phlegm was thought to be associated with reserved behavior, as preserved in the word *phlegmatic.* The phlegm of humorism is far from the same thing as the phlegm that is defined today.

The system of medicine was highly individualistic, for all patients were said to have their own unique humoral composition.[6]

2.1.2   Changes Initiated by Hippocrates: The Father of Medicine

- Research started to help eliminate superstitions.
- Diseases were caused by the lack of sanitation.
- No dissection, only observations and careful notes of signs/symptoms of diseases.
- Diseases were not caused by supernatural forces.
- Illnesses were the result of natural causes.
- Standard of ethics was written, which is the basis for today's medical ethics.
- One should never cause harm to the patient.
- Aesculapius and the serpent symbol of medicine; temples built in his honor became the first true clinics and hospitals.

2.1.3   Summary and Thoughts on Ancient Medicine

1. The *Sushruta Samhita* (India) is one of the most important surviving ancient treatises on medicine, and Sushruta is considered the main writer of the foundational text of Ayurveda.

2. The term *microscope* was mentioned in different texts during the Roman era, but it was not developed until around 1620, at least not according to the definition we would use today. During ancient times, the term *microscope* could describe something like a magnifying glass. The modern term *microscope* means a set of lenses with both an ocular and an object lens or a combination of lenses.

3. Humorism (i.e., chemical systems regulating human behavior). The theory of humorism was built on a belief that the human body consisted of four different substances called humors and illnesses arose when the balance among the four humors was changed and the relation among the four humors was unbalanced. Consequently, the treatment was to bring back the balance to each of the four humors: blood, yellow bile,

black bile, and phlegm. Human temperaments and personalities were linked to these four humors: cheerful, blood; unemotional, yellow bile; annoyed, black bile; and sad, phlegm. The theory based upon humorism survived many centuries, in fact until the mid-18th century.[7]

4. The belief that diseases and illnesses were caused by demons and evil spirits was still around. Treatment was often directed toward eliminating the evil spirit. As civilization developed, changes occurred; people began studying the body and how it functioned. Religion played an important role; illness was a punishment from the gods, and ceremonies were performed to eliminate evil spirits and restore health.

2.2   Medicine in Ancient Rome (753 BC–AD 476)

Medicine in ancient Rome combined various techniques, using different tools, methodologies, and ingredients. Ancient Roman medicine was highly influenced by Greek medicine but would ultimately have its own contribution to the history of medicine through past knowledge of the *Hippocratic Corpus*, combined with the use of the treatment of diet and regimen, along with surgical procedures. This was most notably seen through the works of two of the prominent Greek physicians, Dioscorides and Galen, who practiced medicine and recorded their discoveries in the Roman Empire. This is in contrast to two other physicians, Soranus of Ephesus and Asclepiades of Bithynia, who practiced medicine both in outside territories and in ancient Roman territory, subsequently. Dioscorides was a Roman army physician, Soranus was a representative of the Methodic school of medicine, Galen performed public demonstrations, and Asclepiades was a leading Roman physician. These four physicians all had knowledge of medicine, ailments, and treatments that were healing, long-lasting, and influential to human history.

Ancient Roman medicine was divided into specializations, such as ophthalmology and urology. To increase their knowledge of the human body, physicians used a variety of surgical procedures for dissection that were carried out using many different instruments, including forceps, scalpels, and catheters.

Roman medicine was highly influenced by the Greek medical tradition. The incorporation of Greek medicine into Roman society allowed Rome to transform into a monumental city by 100 BCE. Like Greek physicians, Roman physicians relied on naturalistic observations rather than on spiritual rituals; but that does not imply an absence of spiritual belief. Tragic famines (starvation) and plagues were often attributed to divine punishment; and appeasement of the gods through rituals was believed to alleviate such events miasma (pollution, bad air, night air) was perceived to be the root cause of many diseases, whether caused by famine, wars, or plague. The concept of contagion was formulated, resulting in practices of quarantine and improved sanitation.

One of the first prominent doctors in Rome was Galen. He became an expert on human anatomy by dissecting animals, including monkeys, in Greece. Due to his prominence and expertise in ancient Rome, Galen became Emperor Marcus Aurelius's personal physician.

The Romans also conquered the city of Alexandria, which was an important center for learning; its Great Library held countless volumes of ancient Greek medical information. The Romans adopted into their medical practices many of the practices and procedures they found in the Great Library.[8, 9]

The caduceus is a winged staff with two snakes wrapped around it (see Figure 2.1). It is also called the rod of Asclepius, a snake-entwined staff, which remains a symbol of medicine today. Asclepius was the son of Apollo and the god of medicine in ancient Greek religion and mythology.

Greek symbols and gods greatly influenced ancient Roman medicine. The caduceus, pictured in Figure 2.1, was originally associated with Hermes, the Greek god of commerce. He carried a staff wrapped with two snakes, known as the caduceus. This symbol later became associated with the Roman god Mercury. Later, in the 7th century, the caduceus became associated with health and medicine due to its association with the azoth, the alchemical universal solvent.

Ancient Greece, 1200–200 BC, was the start of the Hippocratic tradition.

Important standards were set concerning ethics and rules for the doctors to obey.

Massage therapy was introduced, and herbal therapy was continually used. The concept that good diet and cleanliness prevented disease was introduced.

The average life span was 25 to 35 years.

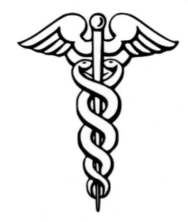

Figure 2.1   The Caduceus. (en.wikipedia.org)[10]

2.2.1 Opposition to Greek Medicine in Rome

In Rome, before there were doctors, the *paterfamilias* (head of the family) was responsible for treating the sick. Cato the Elder himself examined those who lived near him, often prescribing cabbage as a treatment for many ailments, ranging from constipation to deafness. He would issue precise instructions on how to prepare the cabbage for patients with specific ailments. He also used cabbage in liquid form. For example, a mixture of cabbage, water, and wine would be embedded in a deaf man's ear to allow his hearing to be restored. Cato would treat fractured or broken appendages with two ends of a cut reed that were bandaged around the injury.

Many Greek doctors came to Rome. Many of them strongly believed in achieving the right balance of the four humors and restoring the natural heat of patients. Around 200 BC, many wealthy families in Rome had personal Greek physicians. By around 50 BC, it was more common than not to have a Greek physician.

Pedanius Dioscorides (AD 40–90) was a Greek botanist, pharmacologist, and physician who practiced in Rome during the reign of Nero. Dioscorides studied botany and pharmacology in Tarsus. He became a well-known army surgeon for Rome. While traveling with the army, Dioscorides was able to experiment with the medical properties of many plants. Compared to his predecessors, his work was considered the largest and most thorough in regard to naming and writing about medicines; many of Dioscorides's predecessors' works were lost. Dioscorides wrote a five-volume encyclopedia, *De Materia Medica*, which listed over 600 herbal cures, forming an influential and long-lasting pharmacopeia. *De Materia Medica* was used extensively by doctors for the following 1,500 years. Within his five books, Dioscorides mentions approximately 1,000 simple drugs. Also contained in his books, Dioscorides refers to opium and mandragora as sleeping potions that can be used as a natural surgical anesthetic.

Soranus of Ephesus was a Greek physician, born in Ephesus, who lived during the reigns of Trajan and Hadrian (AD 98–138). According to the *Suda*, he trained at the medical school in Alexandria and practiced in Rome. Soranus was a part of the Methodist school of Asclepiades, which fostered the ideals of the Hippocratic doctrine. He was the chief representative of the Methodic school of physicians. Soranus's most notable work was his book *Gynecology*, in which he discussed many topics that are considered modern ideas, such as birth control, pregnancy, midwife's duties, and post-childbirth care. His treatise *Gynecology* is extant (first published in 1838, later by V. Rose in 1882, with a 6th-century Latin translation by Muscio, a physician of the same school). He accounts for the internal difficulties that could arise during labor from both the mother and the fetus. He also did work with fractures, surgery, and embryology.[11]

2.3   Galen of Pergamon (AD 129–216)

Galen (see Figure 2.2) was a Greek who became the Roman Empire's greatest physician, authoring more books still in existence than any other ancient Greeks: About 20,000 pages of his work survived. He was the personal physician to Rome's emperors for decades. Galen had great expertise in anatomy, surgery, pharmacology, and therapeutic methods. He is famous for bringing philosophy into medicine—although most of his philosophical works have been lost. Galen's medical doctrine dominated the Western and Arab worlds for close to 1500 years. He was a prominent Greek physician, whose theories dominated Western medical science for well over a millennium. By the age of 20, he had served for four years in the local temple as a therapist (attendant or associate) of the god Asclepius.

Although Galen studied the human body, dissection of human corpses was against Roman law, so instead, he used pigs, apes, sheep, goats, and other animals. Through studying animal dissections, Galen applied his animal anatomy findings and developed a theory of human anatomy. Galen moved to Rome in 162. There, he lectured, wrote extensively, and performed public demonstrations of his anatomical knowledge. He soon gained a reputation as an experienced physician, leading to attracting many patients to his private practice. Among them was the consul Flavius Boethius, who introduced

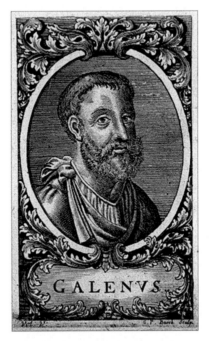

Figure 2.2   Galen of Pergamon. (en.wikipedia.org)[12]

him to the imperial court, where he became a physician to Emperor Marcus Aurelius. Despite being a member of the court, Galen reputedly avoided Latin and spoke and wrote in his native Greek. The Greek language was rather popular in Rome at this time. He treated Roman luminaries, such as Lucius Versus, Commodus, and Septimius. In AD 166, Galen returned to Pergamon but went back to Rome for good a few years later.

Galen followed Hippocrates's theory of the four humors, believing that one's health depended on the balance among the four main fluids of the body (blood, yellow bile, black bile, and phlegm). Food was believed to be the initial object that allowed the stabilization of these humors. By contrast, drugs, venesection, cautery (healing of wounds by burning the surrounding tissue), and surgery were drastic and were to be used only when diet and regimen did not help anymore. The survival and amendment of Hippocratic medicine are attributed to Galen, who coupled the four qualities of cold, heat, dry, and wet with the four main fluids of the body, which would remain in healthcare for a millennium or more.

Galen wrote a short essay called "The Best Doctor Is Also a Philosopher," where he wrote that a physician needs to be knowledgeable about not just the physical but, additionally, logical and ethical philosophy. He wrote that a physician "must be skilled at reasoning about the problems presented to him, must understand the nature and function of the body within the physician world, and must practice temperance and despise all money." The ideal physician treats both the poor and elite fairly and is a student of all that affects health.

Galen thought that eleven years of study was an adequate amount of time to make a competent physician. He references Hippocrates throughout his writings, saying that Hippocratic literature is the basis for physicians' conduct and treatments. The writings of Galen survived longer than the writings of any other medical researchers of antiquity.[12]

2.4   Romans (1200 BC–AD 410)

Summary

- Rooms in doctors' houses where they cared for soldiers became the first hospitals.
- The Romans believed that the body was regulated by four humors that had to stay balanced to prevent illness (blood, phlegm, black bile, and yellow bile).
- The Romans established the first public health and sanitation systems by building sewers and aqueducts.
- The Romans treated diseases with diet, exercise, and medication.
- The Romans realized that some diseases were connected to filth, contaminated water, and poor sanitation.
- They began the development of sanitary systems.

- The Romans built sewers to carry away waste and aqueducts to deliver clean water.
- They also drained swamps and marshes to reduce malaria.
- The Romans also established the first hospital for injured soldiers.
- The Romans learned from the Greeks and developed a sanitation system, aqueducts, sewers, and public baths, and started public health.
- Public hygiene: Food control and solid construction of homes.
- Medicine was practiced only in convents and monasteries.
- Custodial care, life, and death were in god's hands.
- Terrible epidemics: Bubonic Plague (Black Death), smallpox, diphtheria, syphilis, measles, typhoid fever, and tuberculosis.
- Crusaders spread diseases.
- Cities became common.
- Special officers dealt with sanitary problems.
- Realization of the fact that diseases are contagious: Quarantine laws passed.

2.5   Asclepiades of Bithynia (124–40 BC)

Asclepiades studied to be a physician in Alexandria and practiced medicine in Asia Minor as well as Greece before he moved to Rome in the 1st century AD. His knowledge of medicine allowed him to flourish as a physician. Asclepiades was a leading physician in Rome and was a close friend of Cicero.

He developed his own version of the molecular structure of the human body. Asclepiades's atomic model contained multishaped atoms that passed through bodily pores. These atoms were round, square, or triangular. Asclepiades noted that if the atoms were flowing freely and continuously, then the health of the human was maintained. He believed that if the atoms were too large or the pores were too constricted, then illness would present in multiple symptoms, such as fever, spasms, or in more severe cases, paralysis.

Asclepiades strongly believed in hot and cold baths as a remedy for illness; his techniques purposely did not inflict severe pain upon the patient. Asclepiades used techniques with the intent to cause the least amount of discomfort while continuing to cure the patient. His other remedies included listening to music to induce sedation and consuming wine to cure headaches and fevers. Asclepiades is the first documented physician in Rome to use massage therapy.[13]

2.6   Greek Ancient Medicine (1200–200 BC)

They made observations about the human body and the effects of diseases that led to modern medical sciences believing illness is a result of natural causes.

They developed a standard of ethics still used today—the Hippocratic Oath. Hippocrates is called the father of medicine.

Records created by him and other physicians helped to establish that disease is caused by natural causes, not supernatural spirits and demons. The Greeks were the first to stress a good diet and cleanliness to prevent disease. They also used therapies, such as massage, art therapy, and herbal treatments.[14]

2.6.1   The Byzantine Empire

The Byzantine Empire, also referred to as the Eastern Roman Empire, or Byzantium, was the continuation of the Roman Empire in its eastern provinces during Late Antiquity and the Middle Ages, when its capital city was Constantinople. It survived the fragmentation and fall of the Western Roman Empire in the 5th century AD and continued to exist for an additional thousand years until it fell to the Ottoman Empire in 1453. During most of its existence, the empire was the most powerful economic, cultural, and military force in Europe.

Byzantine Empire is a term created after the Ottoman Empire took over in 1453. Its citizens continued to refer to their empire simply as the Roman Empire or Romania and to themselves as Romans. Nevertheless, the Roman state continued, and its traditions were maintained even if it was centered around Constantinople and, hence, oriented toward Greek rather than Latin culture. Several events from the 4th to 6th centuries mark the period of transition during which the Roman Empire's Greek East and Latin West diverged. Constantine I (r. 324–337) reorganized the empire, made Constantinople the new capital, and legalized Christianity.

Under Theodosius I (r. 379–395), Christianity became the state religion, and other religious practices were prescribed. In the reign of Heraclius (r. 610–641), the empire's military and administration were restructured, and Greek was adopted for official use in place of Latin.

The borders of the empire fluctuated through several cycles of decline and recovery. During the reign of Justinian I (AD 527–565), the empire reached its greatest extent, after reconquering much of the historically Roman western Mediterranean coast, including North Africa, Italy, and Rome, which it held for two more centuries. During the Macedonian dynasty (10th–11th centuries), the empire expanded again and experienced the two-century-long Macedonian Renaissance, which came to an end with the loss of much of Asia Minor to the Seljuk Turks after the Battle of Manzikert in 1071. This battle opened the way for the Turks to settle in Anatolia. The empire recovered during the Komnenian restoration, and by the 12th century, Constantinople was the largest and wealthiest city in Europe.

The empire was delivered a mortal blow during the Fourth Crusade when Constantinople was sacked in 1204, and the territories that the empire formerly governed were divided into competing Byzantine Greek and Latin realms. Despite the eventual recovery of Constantinople in 1261, the Byzantine Empire remained only one of several small rival states in the area for the final two centuries of its existence. Its remaining territories were progressively annexed by the Ottomans in the Byzantine–Ottoman wars over the 14th and 15th centuries. The fall of Constantinople to the Ottoman Empire in 1453 ended the Byzantine Empire.[15, 16]

Reference List, Chapter 2

1 https://bmcr.brynmawr.edu/2011/2011.08.37/
2 https://en.wikipedia.org/wiki/Aristotle
3 https://en.wikipedia.org/wiki/Hippocratic_Oath
4 https://en.wikipedia.org/wiki/Alcmaeon_of_Croton
5 www.wikiwand.com/en/Alcmaeon
6 http://en.wikipedia.org/wiki/Humorism
7 https://en.wikipedia.org/wiki/Medical_Renaissance
8 Nicola Barber: *Renaissance Medicine*. Express Edition, Raintree, 2013.
9 www.worldhistory.org/article/207/what-happened-to-the-great-library-at-alexandria/
10 https://en.wikipedia.org/wiki/Caduceus
11 https://sv.wikipedia.org/wiki/Pedanius_Dioskorides
12 https://en.wikipedia.org/wiki/Galen
13 https://en.wikipedia.org/wiki/Asclepiades_of_Bithynia
14 www.worldhistory.org/Greek_Medicine/
15 https://en.wikipedia.org/wiki/Medicine_in_ancient_Rome#cite.
16 https://en.wikipedia.org/wiki/Byzantine_Empire

3

MEDIEVAL MEDICINE (AD 400–1400)

3.1 Medicine and the Church

In medieval times, illness was believed to be a punishment for sins, and God was reckoned to be the divine physician who sent sickness or healing, depending on his will. Consequently, medical treatment was more concerned with caring for the sick, especially their souls, than with curing them. Therefore, when the Roman Catholic Church stated that illness was a punishment from God and that those who were ill were so because they were sinners, few dared to argue.

Certain men of the Church even thought that healing the sick was against God's will and, thereby, endangering the patient's soul. After all, the patient had to pay for the sins he had committed. The healer was also challenged by going against God's will as his own soul was at risk.

Luckily, there were also people that thought that if a cure for a disease was available, then God would have used it. It is clear that during the Medieval Period, medicine could be both controversial as well as complicated.

For a big part of the population, the best way to stay healthy was to avoid diseases and sickness, to prevent it. From the Roman Catholic Church's point of view, this was best done by following the recommendations from the Church by praying and living a holy lifestyle.

Seen from this perspective, it is easy to understand why the Church, no matter what religion we are talking about, kept a very strong impact on the people's everyday life.[1]

3.2 Background of the Early Days of the Middle Ages

The early Middle Ages, or Dark Ages, started when invasions divided Western Europe into small territories run by feudal lords.

After the fall of the Roman Empire, the study of medicine stopped. Individuals lived with little or no personal hygiene. Epidemics of smallpox, typhus, and plague were rampant. Monks and priests stressed prayer to treat illness and disease.

Most people lived in rural servitude. Even by the year 1350, the average life expectancy was 30–35 years, and one in five. There were no services for public health or education at this time, and communication was poor.

DOI: 10.1201/9781003393320-4

Scientific theories had little chance to develop or spread. Only in the monasteries was there a chance for learning and science to continue. Around 1066 CE (Common Era, Gregorian calendar), things began to change. The Universities of Oxford and Paris were established. Monarchs became owners of more territory, their wealth grew, and their courts became centers of culture. Learning started to take root.

Trade grew rapidly after 1100 CE, and towns were formed. However, with them came new public health problems.[2]

In Medieval Europe and its nearby vicinity, the dominating ideas were the ideas from antiquity on how health should be kept and how to get it back in case of disease. Medically competent persons were often nuns and monks, which is exemplified by the universal genius Hildegard of Bingen (1098–1179).

In the monasteries, the nuns and monks translated books written by Greek and Arab medically competent people. At the same time, the knowledge and traditions, like humorism (the theory about the relation among the four different body fluids), almost no doctors did challenge the humorism theory and the need for balance among the different body fluids as a need for good health.

Diseases were believed to be cured by establishing the balance among the four body fluids. The therapy consisted of blood depletion or other types of draining. It was accomplished with a knife or by using a leech (bloodsucking animal). The possible pharmaceuticals used at this time were herbs and roots as well as diuretic aperients and pharmaceuticals for vomiting.[3]

3.3   Summary and Thoughts on Medieval Medicine

1. Monks obtained and translated the writings of the Greek and Roman physicians on smallpox, diphtheria, syphilis, and tuberculosis.
2. The status of medicine is very much the same as during the late phase of the Ancient Period.
3. The dominating theory was humorism, with a focus on the four body fluids.
4. The basis for surgery and anatomy improved during the period, but there was still no take-off for this discipline.
5. There was renewed interest in the medical practices of Greeks and Romans. Bubonic Plague killed 75% of the population in Europe and Asia.
6. Medical universities were created.
7. Arab physicians used chemistry to advance pharmacology.
8. Arabs begin requiring physicians to pass examinations and obtain licenses.
9. The study of medicine stopped for over 1,000 years.
10. Medicine was practiced in monasteries and convents.

11. The first medical school opened toward the end of the Middle Ages.
12. Rhazes invented suturing to close wounds.
13. This brought a renewed interest in the medical practices of the Romans and Greeks.
14. Outbreaks of major diseases: smallpox, diphtheria, tuberculosis, typhoid, and malaria. Many of these diseases are nonexistent today due to vaccines and medications.
15. Even by the year 1350, the average life expectancy was still low, 30–35 years, and one in five children died at birth.

The invention of the microscope was a consequence of improved understanding during the Renaissance Period.

Prior to the 19th century, humorism was thought to explain the cause of disease, but it was gradually replaced by the germ (bacteria) theory of disease, leading to effective treatments and even cures for many infectious diseases.

Military doctors advanced the methods of trauma treatment and surgery. Public health measures were developed, especially in the 19th century, as the rapid growth of cities required systematic sanitary measures. Advanced research centers opened in the early 20th century, often connected with major hospitals. The mid-20th century was characterized by new biological treatments, such as antibiotics. These advancements, along with developments in chemistry, genetics, and radiography, led to modern medicine. Medicine was heavily professionalized in the 20th century, and new careers opened to women as nurses (from the 1870s) and as physicians (especially after 1970).

3.4 Black Death: In Europe, from AD 1347 to AD 1770

Black Death, the Plague, and so on hit Europe very severely during the Middle Ages (Figure 3.1). The Plague killed approximately 25 million people, almost a third of the continent's population. It was extremely contagious. The fact that none, including medical experts, in those days knew the origin of the disease, it was impossible to protect each other from being sick. Today, we know that the Plague was due to the bacterium *Yersinia*. During the Middle Ages, there were no antibiotics, and hence, there was no cure.

The situation those days was very different from the recent or current Covid-19 pandemic situation. Not only because Covid-19 is a viral disease, but because of the fact that it is so contagious and has led to the death of a large group of people. Mainly, the elderly with other pre-existing conditions has been hit very hard.

The Plague, Black Death, and Bubonic Plague were the many names for this terrible time that killed 75% of the population of Europe and Asia—47

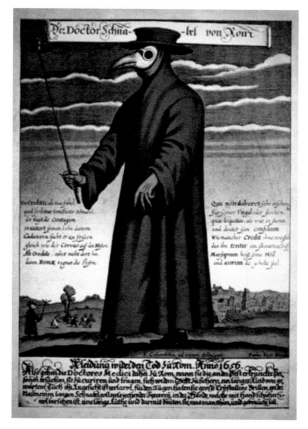

Figure 3.1   A typical drawing representing Black Death from the Middle Ages. (en. wikipedia.org, Black Death)[4]

million people in 10 years. This was transmitted overseas by rats through land and sea travel.

The miasma theory is an old and replaced medical theory that suggested that diseases, like cholera, chlamydia, or the Black Death, were caused by a *miasma* (ancient Greek for "pollution"), a noxious form of bad air; some people called it night air.

The theory held that epidemics were caused by miasma, emanating from rotting organic matter. Though the miasma theory is typically associated with the spread of contagious diseases, some academics in the early 19th century suggested that the theory extended to other conditions as well; for instance, one could become obese by inhaling the odor of food.

The miasma theory was accepted in ancient times in Europe and China. The theory was eventually abandoned by scientists and physicians after 1880 and replaced by the germ theory of disease: Specific germs, not miasma, caused specific diseases. However, cultural beliefs about getting rid of odor made the clean-up of waste a high priority for cities.[5, 6]

3.5   Summary of the Dark Ages (AD 400–800)
and the Middle Ages (AD 800–1400)

1. Terrible epidemics: Bubonic Plague (Black Death), smallpox, diphtheria, syphilis, measles, typhoid fever, and tuberculosis.
2. Crusaders spread disease.
3. Cities became common.
4. Special officers dealt with sanitary problems.
5. Realization that diseases are contagious. Quarantine laws were passed.

Reference List, Chapter 3

1 Toni Mount: *Medieval Medicine. Its Mysteries and Science.* Amberley Publishing, 2016.
2 Faith Wallis: *Medieval Medicine: A Reader.* University of Toronto Press, 2010.
3 https://en.wikipedia.org/wiki/Hildegard_of_Bingen
4 https://en.wikipedia.org/wiki/Black Death
5 Faith Wallis: *Medieval Medicine: A Reader.* University of Toronto Press, 2010.
6 https://en.wikipedia.org/wiki/Miasma_theory 5

4

RENAISSANCE MEDICINE
(AD 1350–1650)

The Renaissance Period stands out against others in history, labeled a cultural rebirth following the Middle Ages. The Renaissance was a fervent period of European cultural, artistic, political, and economic rebirth following the Middle Ages. Generally described as taking place from the 14th century to the 17th century, the Renaissance promoted the rediscovery of classical philosophy, literature, and art.

4.1 The Signature Theory

The Signature theory is a medical theory that dates back to antiquity and means that plants that look like a specific organ in our body have the ability to cure diseases in this specific organ. For example, the leaf of the *Hepatica* flower should be able to cure liver diseases, and the yellow flower will be effective against jaundice. The Signature theory was also recognized in the late 19th-century and early 20th-century alternative medicine and new age teachings. The Signature theory was systemized during the Middle Ages at the pharmacies that started to be established around Europe.

Among the persons that were very engaged in developing the details of the Signature theory was the Middle Ages Swiss doctor Paracelsus. During this era, science and real in-depth knowledge about the human body and its function were built.

Later, you will find a list of scientists that have forever set their name in our history books, as they have made quantum leap contributions to medical and technological developments and science.

4.2 The Age of Discovery (1492–1763)

The period was also called the Age of Exploration and was a period from the early 15th century and continued into the early 17th century, during which European ships traveled around the world to search for new trading routes and partners to feed burgeoning capitalism in Europe. A combination of circumstances stimulated seeking new routes.

There are three main reasons for European exploration. Them being for the sake of their economy, religion, and glory. They wanted to improve their economy, for instance, by acquiring more spices, gold, and better and faster trading routes.

DOI: 10.1201/9781003393320-5

The Age of Discovery did not have any direct impact on medical developments during the Renaissance Period, but it is an important start, enabling future collaborations. Collaboration will be an important step for driving and accelerating medical research forward.

The Covid-19 pandemic that started in early 2020 is an excellent example of how we, today, can develop a vaccine in approximately one year through open global collaboration. In fact, the Age of Exploration was the starting point and enabler for today's fantastic collaboration possibilities that have shown important results when we need these the most.[1]

4.3   Leonardo da Vinci (1452–1519)

Leonardo da Vinci (Figure 4.1) was an Italian painter, draftsman, sculptor, architect, and engineer whose genius, more than anybody else, represented Renaissance humanistic ideals. He is, of course, most famous for his paintings the *Mona Lisa* and the *Last Supper*, plus some of his sculptures, but his impact on the human anatomy through his fantastic sketches must not be forgotten (see Figures 4.2, 4.3, and 4.4).

Leonardo broadened his anatomical work into a comprehensive study of the structure and function of the human organism. The sketches were very important for the knowledge of the coming generations of medical doctors and scientists. Remember, we are 400 years ahead of Roentgen, and anatomy was primarily coming from dissections of cadavers and organs, and many times, from animals.

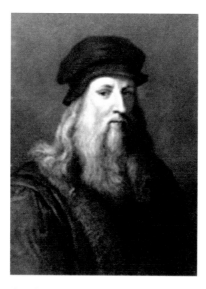

Figure 4.1   Leonardo da Vinci. (en.wikipedia.org, sv.wikipedia.org)[2, 3]

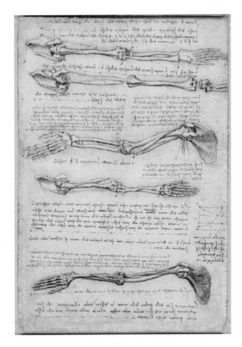

Figure 4.2 Examples of anatomical sketches made at the Hospital of Santa Maria Nuova by Leonardo da Vinci. (sv.wikipedia.org)[4]

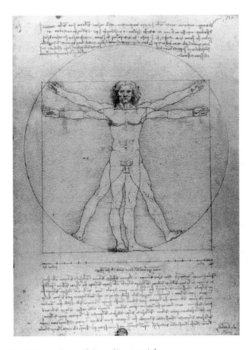

Figure 4.3 *Vitruvian Man.* (sv.wikipedia.org)[4]

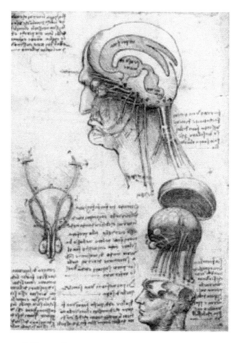

Figure 4.4   Sketches of dissections at the Hospital of Santa Maria. (sv.wikipedia.org)

4.3.1   Most Important Accomplishments

The study of the body was done by dissections.

Leonardo da Vinci and Michelangelo created many inventions and studied and created anatomical drawings.[5]

Ambroise Paré was a French surgeon, anatomist, and inventor of surgical instruments. He was a military surgeon during the French campaigns in Italy (1533–1536). It was here that, having run out of boiling oil (which was the accepted way of treating firearm wounds), Paré turned to an ancient Roman remedy, egg yolk and oil of roses. He applied it to the wounds and found that it relieved pain and sealed the wound effectively. Paré also introduced the ligatures of arteries; the use of silk threads to tie up the arteries of amputated limbs to try to stop the bleeding. As antiseptics had not yet been invented, this method led to an increased fatality rate and was abandoned by medical professionals of the time. Additionally, Paré set up a school for midwives in Paris. He also designed artificial limbs, probably due to his experience as a military surgeon.

4.3.2   Most Important Accomplishments

Paré introduced amputation to the battlefield care of wounded soldiers. He promoted the use of artificial limbs. He introduced the use of ligatures to stop bleeding and bind arteries.[6]

4.4 Andreas Vesalius (1514–1564)

Vesalius broke with the theories of Galen, which at the time still were considered authoritative in medical education, as his own dissections were based on human cadavers, while Galen did not base his anatomy on the dissection of human cadavers, as this was strictly forbidden by the Roman religion. Galen was, therefore, forced to use only animal cadavers for his dissections.

Vesalius started to prepare a comprehensive textbook on human anatomy. Vesalius published his book with the name *De Humani Corporis Fabrica* (*The Seven Books on the Structure of the Human Body*) in 1543.

It is known as the *Fabrica* among medical scientists. After Vesalius, anatomy became a scientific discipline, and the anatomy of the human body became gradually more and more detailed and exact. Vesalius wrote the first anatomy book. The invention of printing made books available to study. Monks were copying books in a monastery prior to the Renaissance.[6]

4.5 Important Developments and Comments on the Renaissance Period (AD 1350–1650)

1. The Signature theory means that plants that look like a specific organ in our body had the ability to cure diseases in this specific organ. Herbs as pharmaceuticals were, therefore, used for curing several diseases. The results were most likely less effective but could maybe alleviate pain or minimize suffering.

2. During this period, the study of human anatomy started to be more solid, as it became systematically based upon human cadavers and organs due to the acceptance of the dissection of the human body during this period. Leonardo da Vinci and Michelangelo used dissection to draw more realistic pictures of the human body. This allowed surgeries to become more precise and led to improved outcomes.

3. The Renaissance was often called the rebirth of the science of medicine. The major source of new information about the human body was a result of accepting and allowing human dissections. Artists such as Michelangelo and Leonardo da Vinci were able to draw the body accurately. Doctors could now view the body's organs and see the connections among different systems in the body.

4. In the 14th to the 16th century, a major epidemic, the Bubonic Plague, killed almost 75% of the population in Europe and Asia. Universities and medical schools for research dissection were established.

5. Book publishing started to be possible, thanks to Johannes Gutenberg's (1400–1468) development of the printing machine/press in 1450.

6. Books could now be published, so universities and medical schools could do more education and research. The first anatomy book, by Andreas Vesalius, was published. This also allowed medical knowledge to be shared with others interested in society.

7. Medical books on the circulatory, respiratory, and digestive systems were released.
8. Gabriele Falloppio (1523–1562) discovered fallopian tubes, connecting the ovaries with the uterus.
9. Bartolomeo Eustachio (1510–1574) discovered the eustachian tube that connects the ear with the throat. He was also the first to give a detailed description of the human hearing organ.
10. Doctors believed that tooth worms caused dental diseases.
11. Antonie van Leeuwenhoek (1676) played with lenses and invented the microscope and started to observe microorganisms.
12. Scientific societies were established.
13. Apothecaries (early pharmacists) made, prescribed, and sold medicines.
14. William Harvey (1578–1657) described the circulation of blood to and from the heart.
15. Girolamo Fracastoro (1483–1553) proposed in the year 1546 that epidemic diseases were caused by transferable seed-like entities. This fact was not proven until much later.
16. Michael Servetus (1511–1553) described the circulatory system in the lungs.

Despite the positive developments previously mentioned, many issues remained to be solved, for example:

• Some quackery (origin is from the Dutch *kwakzalver*) or purveyor of salves were rubbed quickly into the skin.
• The making of health claims without an honest evaluation with usual methods of science was rather common.
• Many died from infection and childbirth fever.

Despite many new discoveries, it did not really create any major changes for ordinary people. The theories from the religious quarters and the Church were still the dominating influence, and most people believed and followed the Church's recommendations. Seen in this way, the Church and religion delayed the development of medicine based on facts and scientific proof.

Reference List, Chapter 4

1 https://en.wikipedia.org/wiki/Age_of_Discovery
2 https://en.wikipedia.org/wiki/Leonardo_da_Vinci
3 https://sv.wikipedia.org/wiki/Leonardo da Vinci
4 Walter Isaacson: *Leonardo da Vinci.* Atlantis, 2018, ISBN: 978-91-7353-987-6, in Swedish.
5 https://pubmed.ncbi.nlm.nih.gov/21560770/
6 https://en.wikipedia.org/wiki/Andreas_Vesalius

5

MEDICINE IN THE 17TH CENTURY (1600–1700)

During the early 17th century, the interest in the anatomy of the human body spread over Europe, and doctors/students were trained in anatomy in many places (Figures 5.1 and 5.2). The Netherlands was probably one of the earliest.

William Harvey (1578–1657) was an English medical doctor/physicist known for his contributions to the heart and blood movement (named physiology today). William Harvey fully believed all medical knowledge should be universal, and he made this his work's goal. Accomplished historians credit him for his boldness in his experimental work and his everlasting eagerness to implement a modern practice. Although not the first to propose pulmonary circulation, he is credited as the first person in the Western world to give quantitative arguments for the circulation of blood around the body. William Harvey's extensive work on the body's circulation can be found in the written work titled *The Motu Cordis*. This work opens with clear definitions of *anatomy* as well as the types of anatomy that clearly outlined the universal meaning of these words for various Renaissance physicians. *Anatomy*, as defined by William Harvey, is "the faculty that by ocular inspection and dissection [grasps] the uses and actions of the parts." In other words, to be able to identify the actions or roles each part of the body plays in the overall function of the body by dissection, followed by visual identification. These were the foundation for further research on the heart and blood vessels.[3]

Nicholas Culpeper (1616–1654) was an English botanist, herbalist, physician, and astrologer. His *The English Physician* (1652; later, *Complete Herbal*, 1653) is a store of pharmaceutical and herbal knowledge, and *Astrological Judgement of Diseases from the Decumbiture of the Sick* (1655) is one of the most detailed works on medical astrology in Early Modern Europe. Culpeper cataloged hundreds of outdoor medicinal herbs.

He did not believe in some of the methods of his contemporaries and expressed his doubts as follows:

> This not being pleasing, and less profitable to me, I consulted with my two brothers, Dr. Reason and Dr. Experience, and took a voyage to visit my mother Nature, by whose advice, together with the help of Dr. Diligence, I at last obtained my desire, and being warned by Mr. Honesty, a stranger in our days, to publish it to the world, I have done it.[59]

DOI: 10.1201/9781003393320-6

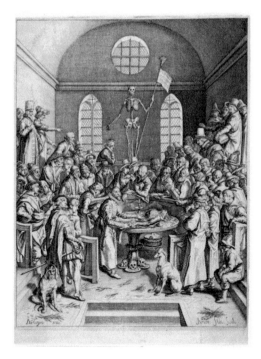

Figure 5.1   Operating theater anatomy. (https://commons.wikimedia.org/
wiki/File:An_anatomical_dissection_by_Pieter_Pauw_in_the_Leiden_anatom_
Wellcome_V0010436.jpg)[1]

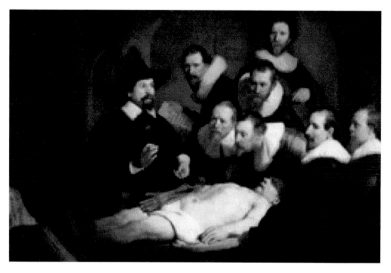

Figure 5.2   Rembrandt van Rijn. The original publication was in 1632, oil on canvas.
(https://en.wikipedia.org/wiki/The_Anatomy_Lesson_of_Dr._Nicolaes_Tulp)[2]

Santorio Santorio (1561–1636), an Italian scientist, is generally credited for having applied a scale to an air thermoscope at least as early as 1612 and, thus, is thought to be the inventor of the thermometer as a temperature-measuring device.[5]

5.1   The Microscope

This is probably one of the most important inventions of all time (Figure 5.3).

Objects resembling lenses date back 4,000 years, and the Greek has evidence of the optical properties of water-filled spheres (5th century BC), followed by many centuries of writings on optics. The earliest known use of simple microscopes (magnifying glasses) dates to the widespread use of lenses in eyeglasses in the 13th century. The earliest known examples of compound microscopes, which combine an objective lens near the specimen with an eyepiece to view a real image, appeared in Europe around 1620. The inventor is unknown, although many claims have been made over the years.

Several revolve around the spectacle-making centers in the Netherlands, including claims it was invented in 1590 by Zacharias Janssen (claims made by his son) and/or Zacharias's father. Hans Martens claims it was invented by their neighbor and rival spectacle maker, Hans Lipperhey (1570–1619),

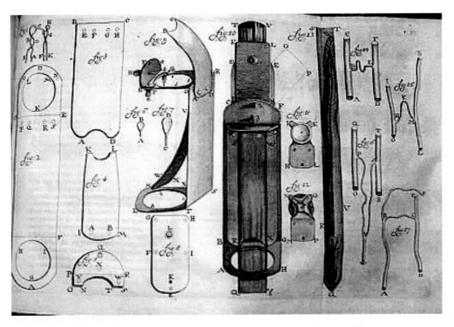

Figure 5.3   Van Leeuwenhoek's microscopes. (en.wikipedia.org)[6]

who applied for the first telescope patent in 1608. Lipperhey claims it was invented by expatriate Cornelis Drebbel, who was noted to have a version in London in 1619.

Despite the many claims of being the inventor of the microscope, the Van Leeuwenhoek microscope was an early version that reached a broader population of users. Galileo Galilei (sometimes cited as the compound microscope inventor as well) seems to have found, after 1610, that he could closely focus his telescope to view small objects and, after seeing the compound microscope built by Cornelis Drebbel (Figure 5.4), exhibited in Rome in 1624, built his own improved version. Giovanni Faber coined the name *microscope* for the compound microscope Galileo submitted to the Accademia dei Lincei in 1625 (Galileo had called it the *occhiolino* or "little eye") (Figure 5.5).

Seen in retrospect, the microscope had a very strong impact on medicine from the very beginning and is one of the most-used instruments in a laboratory presently.

It quickly became the window to see bacteria, which, in turn, had and have a profound importance on many healthcare problems.

Note: A more comprehensive chapter on microscopy will follow, with more modern developments in microscope imaging.[8, 9]

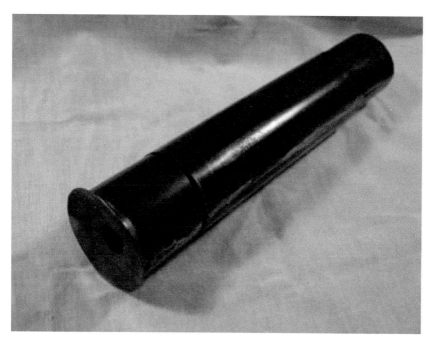

Figure 5.4   Compound microscope probably built by Cornelis Drebbel, exhibited in Rome, 1624. (en.wikipedia.org)[7]

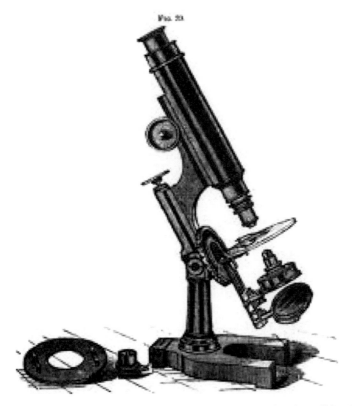

Fig. 51

Figure 5.5   Microscope, looking more like the ones from today. (en.wikipedia.org)[7]

5.2   What Sort of Cures Were Available in the 17th Century?

Chinese people had been using plants for medicinal purposes for 4,500 years, and some of these had been brought to Europe. Many domestic plants, such as foxglove (*Digitalis*) and marsh mallow (*Althea officinalis*), were also used to treat illnesses.

Besides these, doctors believed in the power of powders said to be made from strange ingredients, such as horn from the mythical unicorn and bezoar stone (made famous again in J.K. Rowling's *Harry Potter* books), which was claimed to be the tears of a stag turned to stone. Live worms, fox lungs (for asthma), spider webs, swallow nests, and the skulls of executed criminals were also highly interesting medicinal ingredients.[10]

5.3   Why Did Doctors Use Leeches?

Leeches are a type of slug-like worm used for thousands of years to reduce blood pressure and cleanse the blood. A leech placed on the skin will consume four times its own weight in blood and, with the blood, the toxins that produce diseases. While the leech is sucking, it releases a chemical called hirudin, which prevents coagulation or clotting of the blood.

Fevers were thought to be the result of too much blood in the body: Doctors deliberately cut veins or used leeches to release this bad blood.[11]

5.4   Where Else Were Advances in Medical Treatment Made?

Some advances in medicine came about through treating soldiers and sailors on the battlefield. A Frenchman named Ambroise Paré (1510–1590) discovered that the best way to treat a wound was not to put boiling oil on it, as had previously been the practice, but instead to apply a cold lotion made of egg yolk, oil of roses, and turpentine.

New drugs that became popular included tobacco, coffee, tea, and chocolate: All of them were first used as medicines.

5.6   Was It Easy for Scientists to Investigate the Human Body?

No, it was not easy at all.

The Church in medieval times forbade dissection, the cutting open of dead bodies. This made it difficult for doctors to learn about the workings of the human body. However, in 1543, a surgeon called Vesalius of Brussels published his own illustrated medical manual called *The Fabric of the Human Body*. This was the result of his own secret dissections, and the illustrations were so accurate that they became a very important guide for doctors and surgeons. Even so, progress was slow, and many people had to suffer horrible cures and medicines.

5.7   Important Discoveries Made in the 17th Century
That Helped Improve Doctors' Knowledge

In the 1620s, an Englishman named William Harvey (1578–1657), who had studied at the great Italian medical school in Padua, discovered that blood circulates around in the body, the heart acting as a pump with valves to control the flow.

King Charles I encouraged Harvey's efforts after seeing his work. King Charles II, who came to the throne in 1660 after the death of Cromwell, was also interested in everything scientific, including medicine.[12]

In 1661, a chemist called Robert Boyle (1627–1691) published a book called *The Skeptical Chemist*, which described how the body takes in something from the air to breathe. Boyle also established that without this important gas, which we now know as oxygen, animals and birds would die. In 1662, Charles II granted a Royal Charter to the Royal Society, and this encouraged scientists to attempt new experiments. However, despite such promising developments, many superstitions were still accepted as truths in the 17th century.[13]

5.8   Cesarian Section

The first modern cesarian section was done in 1610 in Germany. The mother survived 24 days while the baby survived much longer.

Already, when Nurma Pompilius (715–672 BC) was the emperor of Rome, the cesarian section was performed in order to save the baby if the woman died late in her pregnancy.

In 1883, the number of cesarian sections documented was 131, while the death rate of mothers was 83%. Most of the mothers died in the early days due to bleeding or infection.

The rate of cesarian sections today in Italy is 40%, while in the Nordic countries, it is only 14%. In the United States, the rate is between 23% and 40%, depending on the actual state.[15, 14]

5.9   What Superstitions Did People Believe In?

Some women who treated people with herbs and potions (drinks that had magical power) were accused of being witches and put to death by hanging or drowning. Another superstitious belief was that the king had the power to cure people of the King's Evil. This was the name given to scrofula or surgical tuberculosis.

The king gave the royal touch on the neck near a gland and gave the sufferer a touch piece or gold coin. This custom dated back to the time of Edward the Confessor (1003–1066).

Charles II may have actually touched, on average, 4,000 persons a year.[16]

5.10   Why Was the Great Plague So Devastating?

In 1665, a plague ravaged England. Lasting from June until November, it reached its peak in September, when in one week, 12,000 people in London died, from a population of around 500,000. The king and his court fled to Oxford, but a doctor named Nathaniel Hodges remained in London to fight the disease. He fumigated houses with smoke from resinous woods, suggested rest and a light diet, and relieved fever by giving his patients Virginia snakeroot. Although his favorite powders were made from bezoar stone, unicorn horn, and dried toad, he found these of no use. He himself sucked lozenges with ingredients of myrrh, cinnamon, and angelica root. Though none of his medicines would have been of any use, he successfully survived in London without contracting the plague.

By the end of the 17th century, a more clinical and scientific approach to health, based on actual observation, gradually began to appear. This laid the foundations for the much greater progress that was to be made in the next century.[17]

5.11   Summary and Thoughts on the 17th Century

1. There was renewed interest in medical practices from the Greeks and Romans.
2. Monks translated from Greek and Roman languages.
3. Leonardo da Vinci drew the body accurately.
4. William Harvey, an English doctor and physicist, is known for his contributions to heart function and blood circulation (today named *physiology*).
5. Antonie van Leeuwenhoek developed the microscope in the year 1676. He began using the lenses to observe the microscopic world. He discovered bacteria, protists, rotifers, and blood cells.
6. Physicians needed to pass examinations to obtain a license.
7. The development of the printing press resulted in the publication of medical books—knowledge spread rapidly.
8. Actual causes of disease were still a mystery.
9. Apothecaries were developed (first pharmacies)—they made, prescribed, and sold medications mostly made from plants and herbs.
10. The Bubonic Plague killed 75% of the population of Europe and Asia.
11. Physicians gained an increased knowledge of the human body. There were improvements in surgical procedures.
12. Blood circulation was discovered.
13. Microscope, mercury thermometer, stethoscope, and bifocals were invented. Benjamin Franklin invented bifocals because he had trouble seeing.
14. Drugstores started to open throughout Europe.
15. Vaccines prevented smallpox.
16. The average life span increased to 30–35 years.

During the 17th century, several new systematic approaches were started and introduced in the field of medicine. Looking back on history, it could be said that a scientific approach to medicine was introduced but did not really reach ordinary people in Europe and Asia. It would take at least another 100 years before ordinary citizens would benefit from the progress made at the top level.[18]

Reference List, Chapter 5

1 https://commons.wikimedia.org/wiki/File:An_anatomical_dissection_by_Pieter_Pauw_in_the_Leiden_anatom_Wellcome_V0010436.jpg
2 https://en.wikipedia.org/wiki/The Anatomy Lesson
3 https://en.wikipedia.org/wiki/William_Harvey
4 www.famousscientists.org/nicholas-culpeper/
5 www.encyclopedia.com/science/encyclopedias-almanacs-transcripts-and-maps/santorio-santorio
6 http://en.wikipedia.org/wiki/Antonie van Leeuwenhoek

7 https://en.wikipedia.org/wiki/Cornelis_Drebbel.

8 www.britannica.com/biography/Galileo-Galilei

9 https://en.wikipedia.org/wiki/Galileo_Galilei

10 www.rmg.co.uk/stories/topics/health-17th-century

11 https://en.wikipedia.org/wiki/Leech

12 https://en.wikipedia.org/wiki/William_Harvey

13 https://en.wikipedia.org/wiki/Robert_Boyle

14 https://en.wikipedia.org/wiki/Caesarean_section#Caesarius_of_Terracina

15 www.hopkinsmedicine.org/health/treatment-tests-and-therapies/cesarean-section

16 https://en.wikipedia.org/wiki/Royal_touch

17 www.history.com/topics/middle-ages/black-death

18 www.rmg.co.uk/stories/topics/health-17th-century

6

MEDICINE IN THE 18TH CENTURY (1700–1800)

The germ theory of disease is the currently accepted scientific theory for many diseases. It states that microorganisms, known as pathogens or germs, can lead to diseases. These small organisms, too small to be seen without magnification, invade humans, other animals, and other living hosts. Their growth and reproduction within their hosts can cause diseases.

A *germ* may refer not just to a bacterium but to any type of microorganism, such as protists or fungi, or even non-living pathogens that can cause diseases, such as viruses and prions. Diseases caused by pathogens are called infectious diseases. Even when a pathogen is the principal cause of a disease, environmental and hereditary factors often influence the severity of the disease and whether a potential host individual becomes infected when exposed to the pathogen.

Basic forms of germ theory were proposed in the late Middle Ages by physicians, including Ibn Sina (980–1037) in 1025, Ibn al-Khatib (1313–1374) in the 14th century, and Girolamo Fracastoro (1476–1553) in 1546, and expanded upon by Marcus von Plenciz (1705–1786) in 1762.[1–3]

However, such views were held in contempt in Europe, where Galen's miasma theory remained dominant among scientists and doctors. He thought that the body was ruled by four humors, or fluids, which determined what your personality was and how you reacted to various diseases.

Seventeenth-century medicine was, unfortunately, still handicapped by wrong ideas about the human body. Very little was known about hygiene in 17th-century England. This was also probably the case in the rest of Europe and the rest of the world.

The impact of hygiene was just not known back then. People were not aware that diseases were spread by germs, which thrived on dirt. They did not think of washing their hands before eating or cleaning the streets, recognizing that diseases could spread quickly due to the environment. People dreaded catching malaria, which they thought came from a poisonous gas called miasma from sewers and cesspits.

6.1 Important Developments during the 18th Century

In 1714, Dutch scientist and inventor Daniel Gabriel Fahrenheit invented the first reliable thermometer, using mercury instead of alcohol and water

DOI: 10.1201/9781003393320-7

mixtures. In 1724, he proposed a temperature scale, which now (slightly adjusted) bears his name.[4]

Sir Charles Bell (1774–1842) was a Scottish surgeon, anatomist, physiologist, neurologist, artist, and philosophical theologian. He is noted for discovering the difference between sensory nerves (a nerve that carries sensory information toward the central nervous system, CNS) and motor nerves in the spinal cord. He is also noted for describing Bell's palsy.[5]

William Withering (1741–1799) was an English botanist, geologist, chemist, and physician, and was the first systematic investigator of the bioactivity of *Digitalis* for the treatment of dropsy/edema (waterfilled organs, like swollen legs).[6]

Samuel Hahnemann (1755–1843) was a German physician and founder of the system of therapeutics known as homeopathy. Homeopathy is a pseudoscientific system of alternative medicine. It was conceived in 1796 by the German physician Samuel Hahnemann. Its practitioners, called homeopaths, believe that a substance that causes symptoms of a disease in healthy people can cure similar symptoms in sick people. All relevant scientific knowledge about physics, chemistry, biochemistry, and biology gained since at least the mid-19th century contradicts homeopathy.[7]

6.2   Summary and Thoughts on the 18th Century

The century was dominated by bringing new ideas, methodologies, and practices into surgery, plus the development of the smallpox vaccine.

1. The development of the microscope and its wider use were key developments, enabling magnifications and possibilities to see bacteria. This led, in turn, to the era of hygiene and steady improvement in surgery methods.
2. The smallpox vaccine was the first vaccine to be developed against a contagious disease. In 1796, the British doctor Edward Jenner demonstrated that infection with the relatively mild cowpox virus conferred immunity against the deadly smallpox virus. Cowpox served as a natural vaccine until the modern smallpox vaccine emerged in the 19th century.
3. William Withering's work on dropsy/edema was important for many surgeries.
4. The development of the stethoscope was an important milestone.
5. Towns with too many people living very close together in a very unhealthy environment due to the lack of any effective sanitary systems, combined with less focus on hygiene, led to many health issues.
6. Public health and hygiene were receiving increased attention during the 18th century.
7. Any medicine that was administered was applied topically to the affected area or dissolved in a liquid-like tea.
8. Life span was 35–45 years.

Reference List, Chapter 6

1 https://en.wikipedia.org/wiki/Avicenna
2 www.wikidata.org/wiki/Q2737184
3 https://en.wikipedia.org/wiki/Marcus_Antonius_Plencic
4 https://en.wikipedia.org/wiki/Daniel_Gabriel_Fahrenheit
5 https://en.wikipedia.org/wiki/Charles_Bell
6 https://en.wikipedia.org/wiki/William_Withering
7 https://en.wikipedia.org/wiki/Samuel_Hahnemann

7

MEDICINE IN THE 19TH CENTURY (1800–1900)

Sir Humphry Davy (1778–1829) was a Cornish chemist and inventor who is best remembered today for isolating, by using electricity, a series of elements for the first time—potassium (K) and sodium (Na) in 1807 and calcium (Ca), strontium (Sr), barium (Ba), magnesium (Mg), and boron (B) the following year—as well as discovering the elemental nature of chlorine (Cl) and iodine (I). Davy also studied the forces involved in these separations, inventing a new field, electrochemistry.

In 1799, Davy experimented with nitrous oxide and was astonished at how it made him laugh, so he nicknamed it the laughing gas and wrote about its potential anesthetic properties in relieving pain during surgery. He also invented the Davy lamp, a very early form of the arc lamp. An arc lamp or arc light is a lamp that produces light using an electric arc.

Nitrous oxide, commonly known as laughing gas or nitrous, is a chemical compound, an oxide of nitrogen with the formula NO. At room temperature, it is a colorless non-flammable gas with a slight metallic scent and taste. At elevated temperatures, nitrous oxide is a powerful oxidizer, like molecular oxygen. In the year 1800, Humphry Davy announced the anesthetic properties of nitrous oxide.[1]

Friedrich Sertürner (1783–1841) was the first to isolate morphine from opium. He called the isolated alkaloid *morphium* after the Greek god of dreams, Morpheus. Sertürner became the first person to isolate the active ingredient associated with a medicinal plant or herb. The branch of science that he originated has since become known as alkaloid chemistry.[2]

Ignaz Philipp Semmelweis (1818–1865) was a Hungarian physician whose work demonstrated that hand-washing could drastically reduce the number of women dying after childbed fever (puerperal fever). This work took place in the 1840s, while he was the director of the maternity clinic at the Vienna General Hospital in Austria. His effort on hand-washing had to begin with very limited effect, as proof was lacking. Doctors were believed to be gentlemen and, therefore, clean. Despite the fact that germ theory had been introduced, the practical introduction in the different medical disciplines took time. The hygiene concept took a long time to become widely accepted. Still today, during the Covid-19 pandemic, it has been hard to make people understand and practice strict hygienic behavior.[3]

DOI: 10.1201/9781003393320-8

James Marion Sims (1813–1883) was an American physician in the field of surgery, both known as the father of modern gynecology and as a controversial figure for the ethical questions raised in developing his techniques.

Sims perfected his surgical techniques by operating without anesthesia on enslaved Black women. In the 20th century, this was condemned as an improper use of human experimental subjects, and Sims was described as "a prime example of progress in the medical profession made at the expense of a vulnerable population." Sims's practices were defended as consistent with the era in which he lived, by physician and anthropologist L. Lewis Wall, and according to Sims, the enslaved Black women were "willing" and had no better option.[4]

Rene Laennec (1781–1826) was a French physician and musician. His skill of carving his own wooden flutes led him to invent the stethoscope in 1816 (Figures 7.1 and 7.2) while working at the Hospital Necker in Paris. He pioneered its usage in diagnosing various chest conditions. He became a lecturer at the Collège de France in 1822 and a professor of medicine in 1823. His final appointments were that of head of the medical clinic at the Hospital de la Charité and professor at the Collège de France. He died of tuberculosis in 1826 at the age of 45.[5]

James Blundell (1790–1878) was an English physician who specialized in obstetrics. In 1818, Blundell proposed that a blood transfusion would be appropriate to treat severe postpartum hemorrhage (today often defined as the loss of more than 500 mL or 1,000 mL of blood within the first 24 hours following childbirth).

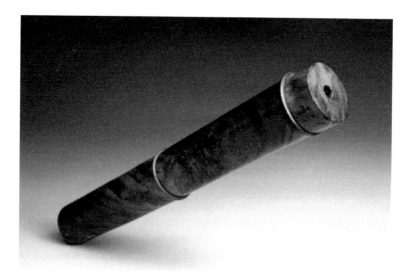

Figure 7.1   Very early stethoscope. (en.wikipedia.org)[5]

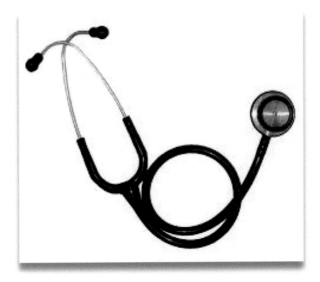

Figure 7.2   Modern stethoscope. (en.wikipedia.org)[5]

He had seen many of his patients dying in childbirth. The most common cause is the poor contraction of the uterus following childbirth. Not all the placenta being delivered, a tear of the uterus, or poor blood clotting are other possible causes.[6]

Crawford Long (1815–1878) was an American surgeon and pharmacist best known for his first use of inhaled sulfuric ether as an anesthetic in 1842 while removing a tumor from the neck of a patient. He administered sulfuric ether on a towel and simply had the patient inhale it.

This was after observing the same physiological effects with diethyl ether (ether) that Humphry Davy had described for nitrous oxide in 1800. After his death, he was officially recognized as the official discoverer of anesthesia.[7]

Joseph Lister (1827–1912) was a British surgeon and a pioneer of antiseptic surgery (Figure 7.3). Lister promoted the idea of sterile surgery while working at the Glasgow Royal Infirmary. Lister successfully introduced carbolic acid (now known as phenol) to sterilize surgical instruments and clean wounds (Figure 7.4).

Before the 1800s, surgery was a risky business. In some London hospitals, the post-operative mortality rates were as high as 80%, and a mortality rate of 50% was considered acceptable. Operations were horrendous ordeals for the patients, with many dying on the table or shortly after from blood loss or post-operative shock. Those that were fortunate enough to survive the procedure then had to run the gauntlet of infection, and because of the limited understanding of how infection was spread at the time, the rate of sepsis was appallingly high.

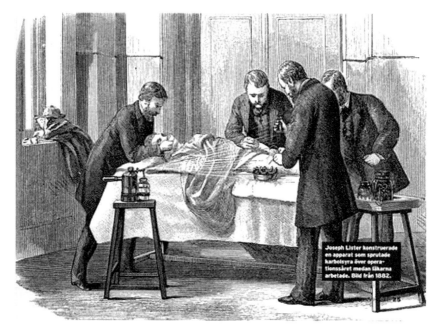

Figure 7.3   Early antiseptic surgery use. Lister during surgery. (en.wikipedia.org)

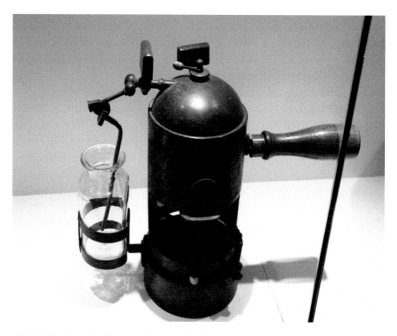

Figure 7.4   Early unit for creating carbolic acid for surgery. (en.wikipedia.org)[8]

In the year 1867, Lister published the *Antiseptic Principle of the Practice of Surgery*, based partly on Louis Pasteur's work.[8]

William Morton (1819–1868) was an American dentist and physician who first publicly demonstrated the use of inhaled ether as a surgical anesthesia in 1846. At the time, physical examination of the patient provided the only clues to the depth of anesthesia. Inexperienced anesthetists could easily overdose the patient. It was not until World War I that the anesthesia community had the first true systematic approach to monitoring.[9]

Robert Liston (1794–1847) was an English surgeon at the University College of London (UCL). He was primarily active before the days of anesthesia, and hence, he had to do his work very fast in order to minimize the duration of pain for his patient.

Liston has been described as "the fastest knife in the West End. He could amputate a leg in 2½ minutes."

His publications include *The Elements of Surgery*, 1831–1832, and *Practical Surgery* in 1837.

Robert Liston, who died very young of an aortic aneurysm in 1847, is chiefly remembered as the first surgeon in Europe to operate under ether anesthesia.[10]

Elizabeth Blackwell (1821–1910) was the first woman to gain a medical degree in the United States, in 1849. The first female medical college in the world was inaugurated in the year 1850 in Philadelphia.[11]

John Hughes Bennett (1812–1875) published the first case of leukemia (1845). "It is moreover the same conclusion which Bennett came to in the much-discussed matter of priority between us when he observed a case of individual leukemia some months before I saw my first case."[12]

Rudolf Virchow (1821–1902), in the year 1858, introduced practical experimental histology and the use of the microscope for the diagnosis of disease into the Scottish medical curriculum. This development put an end to humoral medicine, the theory of the four body fluids.[13]

Louis Pasteur (1822–1895) was a French biologist, microbiologist, and chemist renowned for his discoveries of the principles of vaccination, microbial fermentation, and pasteurization. He is remembered for his remarkable breakthroughs in the causes and prevention of diseases, and his discoveries have saved many lives ever since. He reduced mortality from puerperal fever (also known as childbed fever). Pasteur also created the first vaccines for rabies and anthrax.

His medical discoveries provided direct support for the germ theory of disease and its application in clinical medicine. He is best known to the general public for his invention of the technique of treating milk and wine to stop bacterial contamination, a process now called pasteurization. He is regarded as one of the three main founders of bacteriology, together with Ferdinand Cohn and Robert Koch, and has been called the father of bacteriology and the father of microbiology, though the same appellation has also been applied to Antonie van Leeuwenhoek, the inventor of the microscope.[14]

Robert Koch (1843–1910) was a German physician and microbiologist. As one of the main founders of modern bacteriology, he identified the specific causative agents of tuberculosis, cholera, and anthrax, as well as gave experimental support for the concept of infectious disease, which included experiments on humans and animals.

Anthrax is an infection caused by the bacterium *Bacillus anthracis*. It can occur in four forms: skin, lungs, intestines, and injection. Symptom onset occurs between one day and over two months after the infection is contracted. The skin form presents with a small blister with a surrounding swelling that often turns into a painless ulcer with a black center. The first cholera vaccine developed by Louis Pasteur was on chicken and other animals. This was the first widely used vaccine that was made in a laboratory.[15]

Pierre Paul Émile Roux (1853–1933) was a French physician, bacteriologist, and immunologist. He was one of the very close collaborators of Louis Pasteur and a co-founder of the Pasteur Institute in Paris in 1887.

Virtually all infections with rabies resulted in death until two French scientists, Louis Pasteur and Émile Roux, developed the first rabies vaccination in 1885. Nine-year-old Joseph Meister (1876–1940), who had been mauled by a rabid dog, was the first human to receive this vaccine.[16]

Emil von Behring (1854–1917) was a German physiologist who received the 1901 Nobel Prize in Physiology or Medicine, the first one awarded in that field, for his discovery of a diphtheria antitoxin/serum. He was widely known as the savior of children, as diphtheria used to be a major cause of child death. His work with the disease, as well as tetanus, has come to bring him most of his fame and acknowledgment.[17]

Waldemar Mordecai Haffkine (1860–1930) was a doctor at the Pasteur Institute and was credited for the development of the prophylactic vaccination against cholera and the Bubonic Plague in British India.[18]

Alfred Nobel (1833–1896) was a Swedish chemist, engineer, inventor, businessman, and philanthropist. He is most famous for being the inventor of dynamite and for instituting the Nobel Prize (Figures 7.5 and 7.6). In his will, he bequeathed his fortune to the Nobel Prize institution.

This led to the first yearly Nobel Prize award in 1901. The following science prizes were announced: Physics, Chemistry, Physiology or Medicine, and Literature.

The Swedish Central Bank, *Sveriges Riksbank*, celebrated its 300th anniversary in 1968 by donating a large sum of money to the Nobel Foundation to be used to set up a sixth prize in the field of Economics in honor of Alfred Nobel.[19]

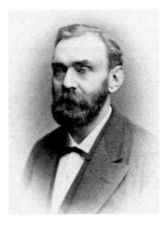

Figure 7.5   Alfred Nobel. (www.wikiwand.com)[19]

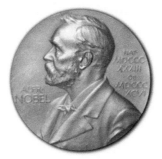

Figure 7.6   Copy of the medal given to each Nobel Prize winner. (www.wikiwand. com)[19]

7.1   The Main Scientific Contributors That Enabled the Introduction of Medical Imaging

Going into the era of medical imaging, there is a need to mention some of the most important inventions and developments that had a strong impact and importance in the coming generations of researchers' possibility to make their scientific contributions to mankind.

The understanding of light was an important piece of knowledge for the 20th century's many developments:

* *Sir Isaac Newton* (1671): Particle model of light.
* *Christiaan Huygens* (1678): Huygens also provided much of the groundwork for the law of conservation of energy, the wave theory of light, and the mathematics of probability.

- *Thomas Young* (1801): Of his many achievements, the most important was establishing the wave theory of light. He proved that light propagates as a wave. He demonstrated interference patterns. The double-slit experiment manifested the principle of duality of the light as a wave and a particle.
- *Augustin Fresnel* (1815): First to propose that light is a wave.
- *James Clerk Maxwell* (1873): The electromagnetic theory.
- *Max Planck* (1897): Electromagnetic radiation is emitted as quanta.
- *Heinrich Hertz* (1889): First to prove the existence of electromagnetic waves.
- *Albert Einstein* (1905): Photon model of light.
- *William David Coolidge* (1913): He invented what would later be known as Coolidge tubes, which create X-rays by using a vacuum tube.
- *Wilhelm Roentgen* (1895): The understanding and discovery of X-rays.
- *Julius Plücker* (1876): He was a pioneer in the investigations of cathode rays that led eventually to the discovery of the electron.
- *Henri Becquerel* (1896): He was a French scientist working along the same lines as Roentgen and discovered a natural radiation source.
- *George Eastman* (1888): Introduction of film.
- *Sir William Morgan*: He was said to be the first experimenter of X-rays, 110 years before they were brought into everybody's mind by Roentgen in 1895.
- *Michael Faraday* (1821): He discovered that a magnetic field influenced polarized light.
- *Wilhelm Hittorf* (1870): He discovered the fluorescent discharge termed cathode rays.
- *J.J. Thompson* (1897): He showed that the cathode ray consisted of negatively charged particles, the electron.

7.2   The Birth of Radiology

Wilhelm Conrad Roentgen (1845–1923) was a German mechanical engineer and physicist (Figure 7.7) who, on November 8, 1895, produced and detected electromagnetic radiation in a wavelength range known as X-rays or Roentgen rays. This achievement earned him the first Nobel Prize in Physics in 1901.

Many researchers and medical doctors have expressed that it was the most important discovery of the 19th century.

Let's describe the experiments that led Roentgen to his discovery.

Wilhelm Conrad Roentgen conducted experiments with cathode ray tubes (*Kathoden-strahlen*). The tubes used were glass bulbs made by a glassblower, with two or more electrical connectors inside the glass bulb as well as a small pump with which it was possible to lower the gas pressure. The gas tubes contained residual gas molecules, as it was not possible to obtain a perfect

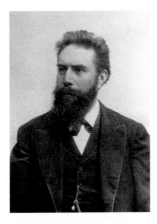

Figure 7.7   Wilhelm Conrad Roentgen. (www.wikiwand.com)[20]

vacuum at this time. Between the anode (+) and the cathode (–), a high voltage was applied (Figure 7.8).

At this time, the particles in the tubes were unknown, but later, it was discovered to be electrons. The electron was not discovered until 1897 by J.J. Thomson.

Roentgen knew that the rays inside the tube were electrically negative, as he could deflect them with a magnet. During the 19th century, observers wondered about the light effects that were emitted from some minerals spontaneously.

Today, we know this light emission as luminescence. There are two types of luminescence: phosphorescence and fluorescence. The difference between the two types is that the phosphorescent material continues to emit light for some time after stimulation, after glowing, while fluorescent material stops glowing very quickly after the radiation source is switched off (Figure 7.9).

Roentgen uncovered a startling effect—namely, that a screen coated with a fluorescent material placed outside a discharge tube would glow even when it was shielded from the direct visible and ultraviolet light of the gaseous discharge.

He deduced that invisible radiation from the tube passed through the air and caused the screen to light up (fluorescence). Roentgen was able to show that the radiation responsible for the fluorescence originated from the point where the cathode rays (electron beam) struck the glass wall of the bulb of the discharge tube. Objects not transparent to light, opaque objects, placed between the tube and the screen proved to be transparent to the new form of radiation.

Roentgen dramatically demonstrated this by producing a photographic image of the bones of the human hand. His discovery of the so-called

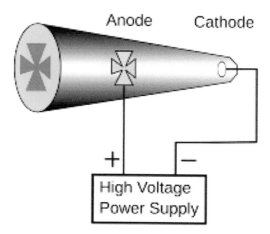

Figure 7.8   The principle of the Crookes tube circuit. (www.wikiwand.com)[21]

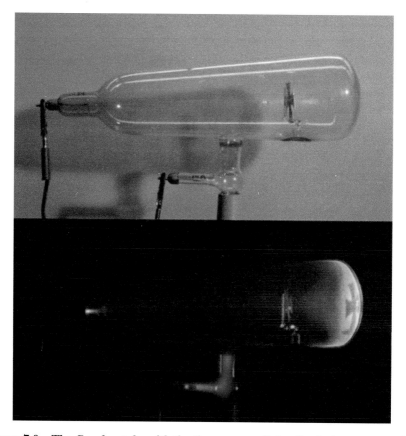

Figure 7.9   The Crookes tube with the fluorescence light after being connected.[22]

Roentgen rays (X-rays) was met with worldwide scientific and popular excitement, and along with the discoveries of radioactivity (1896) and the electron (1897), it jumpstarted the study of the atomic world and the era of modern physics.

7.2.1   Description of the Experiments That Roentgen Conducted When He Discovered X-rays

Roentgen conducted experiments with a so-called Crookes tube, which is a gas tube with remaining gas molecules (i.e., not with a complete vacuum).

When a high voltage is connected between the anode (+) and cathode (–) of the tube, the gas molecules will be split into an electron and a positive ion. The positive ions will go to the cathode, and the electrons will be drawn toward the anode. When the electrons hit the anode, X-rays are generated. In the experiment that Roentgen conducted, the X-rays, in turn, hit a fluorescent material that was available in Roentgen's laboratory (Figure 7.10), and when the X-rays hit the fluorescence powder, it lit up. Roentgen did the experiment on November 8, 1895. Between this date and the date when he first published the paper "On a New Kind of Rays," he did extremely many experiments to verify his original findings in a very impressive systematic way.

Maybe one of the most interesting findings and game-changing experiments was when he investigated the new X-ray's physical properties and held a piece of lead in the beam, and he saw some of his fingers appear on the photographic film he used for documentation.

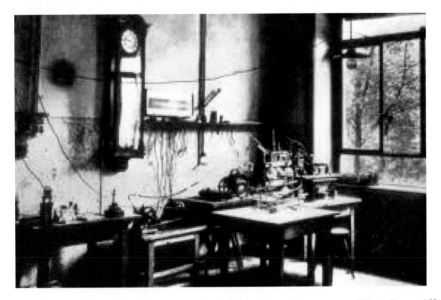

Figure 7.10   Wilhelm Conrad Roentgen's laboratory. (commons.wikimedia.org)[23]

My personal thought is that this was the time he really understood the great potential of the new rays. I saw this X-ray image, several years ago when I visited the Roentgen Museum in Würzburg, where it was for display. Not the highest image quality but very convincing.

The following is the chronological sequence of activities of the investigation of the new X-rays just discovered by Wilhelm Conrad Roentgen:

- December 28, 1895: All the experiments he did in his laboratory were described in the article he submitted with the title "On a New Kind of Rays," as a preliminary communication to the secretary of the Physikalisch-Medizinische Gesellschaft at Würzburg for publication.
- January 1, 1896: Roentgen sent reprints of his preliminary paper to many colleagues in Europe. Some received a set of X-rays with the reprints. An X-ray of the hand of Roentgen's wife, Bertha, was one of the reprints.
- January 5, 1896: *Die Presse* in Vienna published an article about the discovery, and the news was cabled out over the whole world.
- January 13, 1896: Roentgen demonstrated the X-rays to Emperor Wilhelm II and the military staff in Berlin.
- January 23, 1896: Roentgen delivered his only public lecture about X-rays in Würzburg at the meeting of the Physikalisch-Medizinische Gesellschaft. Professor Albert Kölliker recommended calling the rays *Roentgen Strahlen,* after the discoverer, which the audience applauded. After this presentation, Roentgen declined all invitations for presentations.
- March 9, 1896: Roentgen's second communication was sent to the Physikalisch-Medizinische Gesellschaft.
- March 10, 1897: Roentgen submitted his third and final communication on X-rays to the Preussiche Akademie der Wissenschaften in Berlin.
- April 1, 1900: Roentgen accepted the professorship in physics at the University of Munich, Germany.
- December 10, 1901: Roentgen received the first Nobel Prize in Physics.[24]

From the X-ray images below, it is clearly visible how the image quality improved in the two months between the two images of the hands of Mrs. Roentgen (Figure 7.11) and Albert von Kölliker (Figure 7.12), respectively.

It was recognized very early by Roentgen himself that the X-rays had an ionizing potential and, hence, could be dangerous for all biological tissue. Despite the early recognition of the risks of the X-rays, many radiologists were saying that the X-rays were harmless (Figure 7.13).

The introduction worldwide was extremely rapid, and the excitement from the medical community was massive. In less than a year, Roentgen's procedures were spread to almost every country in the world. Although the risks were known, they were neglected or minimized by too many practicing radiologists. The effect was that many radiologists lost their fingers and hair and got radiation-induced cancer.

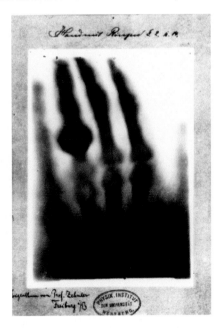

Figure 7.11   X-ray of Mrs. Roentgen's hand, November 1895. (commons. wikimedia.org)[23]

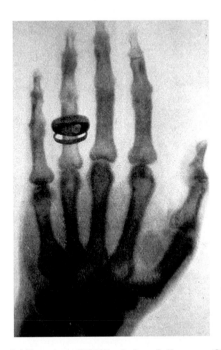

Figure 7.12   X-ray of Albert von Kölliker's hand, January 23, 1896. (commons. wikimedia.org)

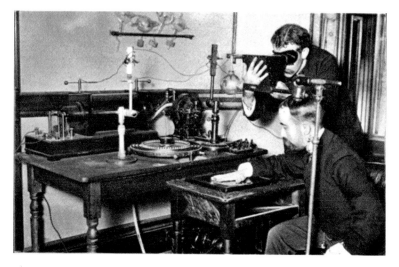

Figure 7.13   Roentgen examination, year 1896. Note that it is totally without radiation protection. (en.wikipedia.org)[24]

Several physicists had, as Roentgen did, seen the same phenomenon of X-rays approximately at the same time, but nobody investigated the full effects of the X-rays as Roentgen did.

Already in his first communication, "On a New Kind of Rays," published February 14, Roentgen reported on a substantial number of measurements and observations with high scientific quality.

The following two communications with additional proof and characteristics of the X-rays were published on March 9, 1897, and October 7, 1897, respectively. These science papers were all he ever published about X-rays. Some scientists have called the X-ray discovery "the birth of radiology" and "the most important discovery of all times."

The impact it had was amazing, as it was a true breakthrough both in the way it was spread immediately and in the way that the news reached all over the world. Consequently, in 1896, X-rays were already produced all over the world.

A good example of how the news about Roentgen's discovery was in Colorado. On February 5, 1896, the *Colorado Springs Gazette* announced the discovery of the X-rays as "The Newest Kind of Photography." Very soon thereafter, the scientists made their own X-rays, as they had a Crooks tube in the laboratory.

New improved X-ray tubes were developed at an accelerating speed. The discovery of X-rays and the very rapid introduction into clinical practice were starting points of a new era with fantastic imaging modalities, one after the other, enabling the diagnosis of almost every disease in the human body.

The sad part of the early developments of the X-ray technique was that the safety aspects of the new rays were not taken very seriously. X-rays are ionizing radiation and, hence, have radiobiology consequences.

Roentgen knew about the safety issues very early, but the excitement, the rapid spread of the technique, and the important impact of being able to see into the human body made the operating personnel of the new X-ray units often forget or avoid using protection during exposure in an imaging session.

Also, early radiologists neglected to protect themselves and lost fingers or got cancer due to imaging with the early X-ray tubes that were without shielding or lacked sufficient shielding and radiation protection.

Let me now give you a physicist's description of the generation of X-rays discovered by Roentgen but with our modern terms and the knowledge we have today.

In the very early days of Roentgen's discovery of the so-called X-rays, the glass tubes used could only be pumped to a rather low pressure, which means that residual gas molecules were left in the tube/glass bulb. This means that when the high voltage was applied between the cathode and the anode, these remaining gas molecules were split into two different populations: One consisted of positive ions that were driven toward the negative pole, the cathode of the tube, and one category was driven toward the positive, namely the electrons.

As we learned how to pump out more or less all gas molecules, the modern X-ray tube could be developed, where the electrons are generated in the cathode by itself via a glowing filament. The electron beam will be driven/accelerated toward the anode by the high tension applied between the cathode and the anode. When the electrons hit the anode, X-rays are generated.[25]

The modern X-ray tube will be discussed later in the book (Chapter 9).

7.3   Summary of the 19th Century

In this century, many developments were about solving important clinical healthcare issues that the whole society would benefit from, like anesthetic and antiseptic surgery, as well as the first human blood transfusion.

Another important step was the introduction of female doctors, led by Elizabeth Blackwell, who was the first woman to receive a medical degree in the United States, in 1849.

In Europe, the first medical school was in Salerno, south of Naples, Italy, in the ninth century. Unfortunately, there are no remnants from this medical school that was located in the Chapel of the Work of Mercy.

More famous and/or well-known was the medical school in Montpellier, Provence, in the south of France, from AD 985. In the United States, the first medical college was inaugurated in Philadelphia, Pennsylvania, USA, in the year 1850.

Puerperal fever (childbed fever) was a devastating disease until a cure was found. It affected women within the first three days after childbirth and progressed rapidly, causing acute symptoms of severe abdominal pain, fever, and debility. Although it had been recognized from as early as the time of the *Hippocratic Corpus* that women in childbed were prone to fevers, the distinct name, puerperal fever, appears in the historical record only in the early 18th century. The development of the stethoscope led to improved possibilities in diagnosing various chest conditions.

The discovery of diphtheria and tetanus antitoxin/serum had a profound impact on reducing child death, as diphtheria used to be a major cause of child death. The antitoxin for prohibiting tetanus has been very important ever since it was developed. Behring won the first Nobel Prize in Physiology or Medicine in 1901 for the development of serum therapies against diphtheria.

The germ theory was an important step in bringing knowledge in order to understand and fight diseases. This was the final step to outdate and kill the theory of the four body fluids, humorism, that originated from the Greek Period and, as such, has survived approximately 2,500 years.

The development of the vaccine for cholera was another important breakthrough that saved many lives.

Probably the most important development of the century was the medical use of the X-rays. To be able to see into the human body without opening it was, of course, a quantum leap that had fantastic follow-ups that we today benefit enormously from.

There are several reasons for the increasing speed of medical and technical development during the 19th century:

- Each new development opened and stimulated new development via the new knowledge gained.
- Increased communication, travel, and sharing of knowledge gave birth to new ideas.
- Medical certification also for women broadened the medical field considerably.

Stay tuned for the 20th century when everything within medical science, healthcare, and medical technology accelerated.

Reference List, Chapter 7

1 https://en.wikipedia.org/wiki/Humphry_Davy
2 https://en.wikipedia.org/wiki/Friedrich_Sertürner
3 https://en.wikipedia.org/wiki/Ignaz_Semmelweis
4 https://en.wikipedia.org/wiki/J._Marion_Sims
5 https://en.wikipedia.org/wiki/René_Laennec#Invention_of_the_stethoscope
6 https://en.wikipedia.org/wiki/James_Blundell_(physician)

7 https://en.wikipedia.org/wiki/Crawford_Long
8 https://en.wikipedia.org/wiki/Joseph_Lister
9 https://en.wikipedia.org/wiki/William_T._G._Morton
10 https://en.wikipedia.org/wiki/Robert_Liston
11 https://en.wikipedia.org/wiki/Elizabeth_Blackwell
12 https://en.wikipedia.org/wiki/John_Hughes_Bennett
13 https://en.wikipedia.org/wiki/Rudolf_Virchow
14 https://en.wikipedia.org/wiki/Louis_Pasteur
15 www.nobelprize.org/prizes/medicine/1905/koch/biographical/
16 https://en.wikipedia.org/wiki/Émile_Roux
17 https://en.wikipedia.org/wiki/Emil_von_Behring
18 www.bbc.com/news/world-asia-india-55050012
19 www.wikiwand.com/en/Alfred_Nobel
20 www.wikiwand.com/en/Wilhelm_Röntgen
21 www.wikiwand.com/en/Crookes—Hittorf_tube
22 https://commons.wikimedia.org/wiki/File:Crookes_tube_two_views.jpg
23 https://commons.wikimedia.org/wiki/Wilhelm_Conrad_Röntgen
24 https://en.wikipedia.org/wiki/X-ray
25 Gerd Rosenbusch, Annemarie de Knecht-van Eekelen: *Wilhelm Conrad Roentgen, The Birth of Radiology*. Springer Biographies, 2019.

Part 2

HEALTHCARE IN MODERN TIMES

8

MEDICINE IN THE 20TH CENTURY (1900–2000): AN ACCELERATED DEVELOPMENT IN MEDICINE AND HEALTHCARE

8.1 Introduction

In this chapter, we will look at an increasing number of new medical and technological developments that we today know and have a very hard time living without. Specifically, when it comes to the many imaging technologies that have revolutionized diagnostic medicine and led to many improvements in therapeutics of earlier impossible-to-treat cases. The different modalities and their specifics will be explained in detail, and their strengths and importance in imaging for today's diagnostics and therapeutics will be exemplified with applications in clinical care in oncology, neurology, and cardiology.

8.2 Important Developments during the 20th Century

8.2.1 Discovery of the Existence of Different Human Blood Types: 1901

Karl Landsteiner (1868–1943) was an Austrian biologist, physician, and immunologist. He distinguished the main blood groups in the year 1900, having developed the modern system of classification of blood groups from his identification of the presence of agglutinins (an agglutinin is a substance in the blood that causes particles to coagulate and aggregate; that is, to change from a fluid-like state to a thickened-mass [solid] state in the blood). In 1937, Landsteiner identified, with Alexander S. Wiener, the Rhesus factor, thus enabling physicians to transfuse blood without endangering the patient's life.

With Constantin Levaditi and Erwin Popper, he discovered the polio virus in 1909.

Landsteiner received, in 1930, the Nobel Prize in Medicine. He was posthumously awarded the Lasker Award in 1946 and has been described as the father of transfusion medicine.[1]

8.2.2 Alzheimer's Disease: 1901

Alois Alzheimer (1864–1915) was a German psychiatrist and neuropathologist who, in 1901, identified and published a paper on the first case describing what is later called Alzheimer's disease.[2]

DOI: 10.1201/9781003393320-10

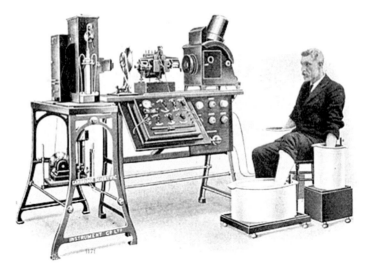

PHOTOGRAPH OF A COMPLETE ELECTROCARDIOGRAPH, SHOWING THE MANNER IN WHICH THE ELECTRODES ARE
ATTACHED TO THE PATIENT, IN THIS CASE THE HANDS AND ONE FOOT BEING IMMERSED IN JARS OF
SALT SOLUTION

Figure 8.1   The very first ECG machine was demonstrated by Willem Einthoven.
(en.wikipedia.org)[3]

8.2.3   Invention of the Electrocardiogram: 1903

Willem Einthoven (1860–1927) was a Dutch physician and physiologist. He invented the first practical electrocardiogram (ECG) equipment in 1901 (Figure 8.1). The equipment was rather bulky, with buckets instead of electrodes. Since they were developed, ECG units have been smaller and very compact. Einthoven received the Nobel Prize in Physiology or Medicine in 1924 for the discovery of the mechanism of the electrocardiogram.[4]

In the period from 1906 to 1927, there were a number of important explanations for specific diseases, together with the development of some important vaccines:

- 1907: Paul Ehrlich develops a chemotherapeutic cure for sleeping sickness.[5]
- 1921: Frederick Banting and Charles Best discover insulin—very important for diabetes patients.[6]
- 1923: First vaccine for diphtheria.[7]
- 1926: First vaccine for pertussis. [7]
- 1927: First vaccine for tuberculosis. [7]
- 1927: First vaccine for tetanus. [7]
- 1935: First vaccine for yellow fever. [7]
- 1938: Howard Florey and Ernst Chain investigate penicillin and attempted to mass-produce it.[8]
- 1952: Jonas Salk develops the first polio vaccine (first available in 1955).[9]

8.2.4   The Discovery of Penicillin: 1928

Alexander Fleming (1881–1955) was a Scottish physician and microbiologist, best known for discovering the enzyme lysozyme and the world's first broadly effective antibiotic substance, which he named penicillin. He received the Nobel Prize in Physiology or Medicine in 1945, together with Howard Florey and Ernst Boris Chain.[10]

8.2.5   Discovery of Vitamins and the Consequence of the Lack of Vitamins: 1906

Frederick Gowland Hopkins (1861–1947) was an English biochemist who was awarded the Nobel Prize in Physiology or Medicine in 1929. He shared the prize with Christiaan Eijkman.[11]

Henry Stanley Plummer (1874–1936) developed the first structured patient record and clinical number (Mayo Clinic) in 1907.[12]

8.2.6   New Surgery Methods in Combination with Technical Tools for Improving Outcomes

During the 20th century, many new surgery methods were developed. Several of these had a major impact on many patients around the world and have continuously been improved ever since. Most of these surgery methods did not have any or very little technology development attached as they were introduced, but new technical tools and instruments quickly followed.

The development of improved anesthesia techniques and chemicals improved the situation for successful and painless surgery:

- 1908: Victor Horsley and R. Clarke invented the stereotactic method. Stereotactic refers to precise positioning in three-dimensional space. For example, biopsies, surgery, or radiation therapy can be done stereotactically.[13]
- 1909: Richard Richter described the first intrauterine device.[14]
- 1910: Hans Christian Jacobaeus performed the first laparoscopy on humans. Laparoscopy is a surgical procedure in which a fiber optic instrument is inserted through the abdominal wall to view the organs in the abdomen or permit small-scale surgery.[15]
- 1917: Julius Wagner-Jauregg discovered the malarial fever shock therapy for general paresis of the insane.[16]
- 1921: Edward Mellanby discovered vitamin D and showed that its absence causes rickets.[17]
- 1929: Hans Berger discovered human electroencephalography.[18]
- 1930: First successful sex gender reassignment surgery was performed, male to female, on Lili Elbe in Dresden.[19]
- 1932: Gerhard Domagk developed a chemotherapeutic cure for streptococcus.[20]

- 1933: Manfred Sakel discovered insulin shock therapy.[21]
- 1935: Ladislas J Meduna discovered metrazol shock therapy.[22]
- 1936: Egas Moniz discovered prefrontal lobotomy for treating mental diseases.[23]
- 1936: Enrique Finochietto developed the new ubiquitous self-retaining thoracic retractor, a mechanical tool used for large-area surgeries.[24]
- 1938: Ugo Cerletti and Lucio Bini discovered electroconvulsive therapy (ECT).[25]
- 1947: Albert Salman X-rayed mastectomy samples and found differences between cancerous and normal tissues.[26]
- 1932: Carl D. Anderson and Robert Millikan began cosmic-ray studies that led to the discovery of the positron.[27]
- 1932: Ernest Lawrence invented the cyclotron for the production of radioactive substances.[28]
- 1953: Gordon L. Brownell invented the technology that evolved into positron-emission tomography (PET).[29]

8.2.7 The Dialysis Machine: 1943

Willem Johan "Pim" Kolff (1911–2009) was a pioneer of hemodialysis, artificial heart, as well as in the entire field of artificial organs. Willem was a member of the Kolff family, an old Dutch patrician family. He made his major discoveries in the field of dialysis for kidney failure during World War II, in 1943.

Willem Kolff has been called the father of artificial organs.[30]

8.2.8 The Disposable Plastic Endotracheal Tube: 1944

David S. Sheridan (1908, Brooklyn–2004, Argyle New York) was the inventor of the disposable plastic endotracheal tube.[31]

8.2.9 The Defibrillator: 1947

Claude Schaeffer Beck (1894–1971) was a pioneer American cardiac surgeon, famous for innovating various cardiac surgery techniques and performing the first defibrillation in 1947.[32]

8.2.10 The Release and Reuptake of Catecholamine Neurotransmitters: 1948

Julius Axelrod (1912–2004) was an American biochemist. He won a share of the Nobel Prize in Physiology or Medicine in 1970, along with Bernard Katz and Ulf von Euler. The Nobel Committee honored him for his work on the release and reuptake of catecholamine neurotransmitters, a class of chemicals in the brain that include epinephrine, norepinephrine, and as was later discovered, dopamine.

Axelrod also made major contributions to the understanding of the pineal gland and how it is regulated during the sleep–wake cycle.

Julius Axelrod, together with Bernard Brodie, was also involved in the verification of the drug paracetamol for pain reduction. It is still today a drug that is very common and used by many people around the world and, hence, a drug with a huge market.[33]

8.2.11   Chemotherapy: 1946

Alfred Goodman Gilman (1941–2015) was an American pharmacologist and biochemist. He and Martin Rodbell (1925–1998), an American biochemist and endocrinologist, shared the 1994 Nobel Prize in Physiology or Medicine "for their discovery of G-protein and the role of these proteins in signal transduction in cells."

G-proteins, also known as guanine nucleotide-binding proteins, are a family of proteins acting as molecular switches inside cells and are involved in transmitting signals from a variety of stimuli outside a cell to its interior.[34]

8.2.12   The Intraocular Lens: 1949

Harold Lloyd Ridley (1906–2001) was an English ophthalmologist who invented the intraocular lens and pioneered intraocular lens surgery for cataract (cloudy lens) and myopia (nearsightedness) patients.[35]

8.2.13   The Iron Lung

John Haven "Jack" Emerson (1906–1997) was an American inventor of biomedical devices, specializing in respiratory equipment. He is perhaps best remembered for his work in improving the iron lung.[36]

8.2.14   Genetics

At the beginning of the 1950s, several research projects around the world were ongoing, with an attempt to explain how genetics was built. It was known that some proteins are entwined in some sort of chains and that the DNA (deoxyribonucleic acid) is carrying genetic information. James Watson (1928–2018) and Francis Crick (1916–2004) published in April 1953, in the scientific journal *Nature*, three back-to-back articles on the structure of DNA, the material our genes are made of. The double-helix structure was verified by using X-ray crystallography.

Together, they constituted one of the most important scientific discoveries in history.

The first purely theoretical article was written by Watson and Crick from the University of Cambridge. Immediately following this article were two data-rich papers by researchers from King's College London: One was by Maurice Wilkins (1916–2004) and two colleagues; the other was by Rosalind Franklin and a PhD student, Ray Gosling.

In 1962, James Watson, Francis Crick, and Maurice Wilkins received the Nobel Prize in Physiology or Medicine for their work on the structure of the DNA molecule. Rosalind Franklin and Ray Gosling's contribution was forgotten.

There is a Nobel Prize stipulation that states, "in no case may a prize amount be divided between more than three persons." The fact she died before the prize was awarded may also have been a factor, although the stipulation against posthumous awards was not instated until 1974.[37]

8.2.15   Cloning: 1952

Joachim August Wilhelm Hämmerling (1901–1980) was a Danish German biologist who determined that the nucleus of a cell controls the development of organisms. His experimentation with the green algae *Acetabularia* provided a model subject for modern cell biological research.[38]

Robert Briggs (1911–1983) and Thomas J. King (1921–2000) were two American biologists who experimented with cloning. They showed in 1952 that if only the nucleus was transplanted from the same species as the egg cytoplasm, then only the egg will cleave and can develop into a normal embryo and further into a tadpole.

Cloning is the process of producing individuals with identical or virtually identical DNA, either naturally or artificially. In nature, many organisms produce clones through asexual reproduction. Cloning in biotechnology refers to the process of creating clones of organisms or copies of cell biology via DNA fragments (molecular cloning).[39]

8.2.16   The Heart-Lung Machine

John Heysham Gibbon (1903–1973) was an American surgeon best known for inventing the heart-lung machine in 1953 and performing subsequent open-heart surgeries, which revolutionized heart surgery in the 20th century.[40]

8.2.17   Medical Ultrasonography: 1953

Inge Gudmar Edler (1911–2001) was a Swedish cardiologist who, in collaboration with Carl Hellmuth Herz (1920–1990), a German Swedish physicist, Professor at Lund University, Sweden, developed medical ultrasonography and echocardiography (*ultrasound* is the short and modern name). They became famous because their ultrasound machine could image the mitral valve, the valve between the left atrium and left ventricle of the heart. This led to the capability to replace the mitral valve. Today, mitral valve replacement is a minimally invasive procedure and not an open-heart surgery procedure.[41]

8.2.18   The First Human Kidney Transplant: 1953

Joseph Murray (1919–2012) was an American plastic surgeon who performed the first successful human kidney transplant on identical twins on December 23, 1954. Murray shared the Nobel Prize in Physiology or Medicine in 1990 with E. Donnall Thomas for their discoveries concerning organ and cell transplantation in the treatment of human disease.[42]

8.2.19 Takeaways from the First Half of the 20th Century

Developments of specific tools, drugs, and vaccines for very specific health conditions and diseases.

The rapid progress of medicine in the 20th century was reinforced by the enormous improvements in communication among scientists throughout the world. Through publications, conferences, and later in the century, computers and electronic media, it was possible to connect instantly with the whole world.

Teamwork started to become the new standard, and consequently, it became more difficult to ascribe a specific accomplishment to a particular individual. Results had to be normally credited to more than a single individual.

The medical and technological developments during the first half of the 20th century happened in many different areas by specialists in several different fields. Looking at specific topics, the picture that appears is that they represented solutions to help very specific diseases and/or health problems related to a specific organ in the human body.

The many new vaccines developed for large population groups had a huge impact around the world. The impact of the development of the antibiotic penicillin by Alexander Fleming also had a strong impact on helping patients to survive very tough infections.

The development of the dialysis machine meant that many people with kidney problems could not only survive but even live a rather normal life.

Likewise, the discovery of insulin opened up the revolution within diabetes treatment.

Many new surgery techniques became available due to the improved anatomy knowledge but more so via the functional understanding of the human body.

It is worth mentioning some of the technological developments that opened very advanced surgery methods, like laparoscopy, a minimally invasive surgery method; the stereotactic method; and open-heart surgery, with the help of the heart-lung machine.

Very early in the 20th century, the important discovery of the different human blood types came. This was extremely important in surgeries where the patients lost blood and needed a blood transfusion. This new knowledge meant far fewer complications in connection with blood transfusions.

A development that maybe did not, at first sight, look very spectacular was the existence of vitamins. This turned out to be very important, as lacking some vitamins could have a severe impact on many organs in the human body. The discovery of vitamin D has built the knowledge that lacking vitamin

D can have an impact on osteoporosis, especially for elderly people and for kids when the skeleton is growing and can create rickets or weak bones.

Many clinical discoveries and developments were done and obtained without direct collaboration between clinical researchers and technical or physicist competencies during the early phase of the development.

Very soon, this would change, and different experts will start working closely together in teams in order to solve clinical challenges.

From around the 1970s, it became more and more common to build multidisciplinary research teams in order to solve a clinically challenging question or develop new methods.

Looking ahead, this will become even more important and needed, as it was realized how fantastic and complicated the human organism and its functions are.

The discovery that each cell in the human body contains a complete set of genetic instructions is probably the most fantastic discovery in the 20th century. As our knowledge has been growing in the field of genetics, we start to see fantastic and revolutionary potentials to diagnose and treat most diseases we could not have dreamt of earlier.

New methods are introduced at an earlier, never realized speed. This was enabled, as our in-depth knowledge grew faster and faster.

Combinations of methods and technologies are enabling new diagnostic methods so sensitive and specific that we will be able to cure patients just because of early diagnosis. Therefore, it will be possible to start early treatment and, hence, be less harmful to the patient.

Maybe the most forward-looking discovery was cloning, by Robert Briggs and Thomas King, in 1952, which, in turn, leaned on the experiments done by Joachim Wilhelm Hämmerling. The nucleus of a cell controls the development of the organisms. He experimented with the green algae *Acetabularia* and provided a model subject for modern cell biological research. These works were, in my mind, the foundation and the opening for genetic work milestones to come later in the 20th century and that forever will change the way we look at the world and ourselves as human beings.

8.3   Second Half of the 20th Century

8.3.1   *The Ventouse (Vacuum Extraction): 1954*

Tage Malmström (1911–1995), a Swedish professor, developed the ventouse, the Malmström extractor, in 1954. Originally made with a metal cap, new materials, such as plastics and siliconized rubber, have improved the design so that it is now used more than forceps. Vacuum extraction (VE), also known as ventouse, is a method to assist in the delivery of a baby using a vacuum device. It is used in the second stage of labor if it has not progressed adequately. It may be an alternative to forceps delivery and cesarean section. It cannot be used when the baby is in the breech position or for premature births. The use of vacuum extraction is generally safe, but it can occasionally have negative effects on either the mother or the child.[43]

8.3.2   Tetracycline: 1955

Lloyd Hillyard Conover (1923–2017) was an American chemist and the inventor of tetracycline.

For this invention, he was inducted into the National Inventors Hall of Fame. Conover was the first to make an antibiotic by chemically modifying a naturally produced drug in 1955. Tetracyclines have a broad spectrum of antibiotic action. Originally, they possessed some level of bacteriostatic activity against almost all medically relevant aerobic and anaerobic bacteria.[44]

8.3.3   Electroencephalography Topography: 1957

William Grey Walter (1923–2017) was an American-born British neurophysiologist and cybernetician, who worked with robots and invented the brain electroencephalography (EEG) topography in 1957.

Topographic EEG analysis includes different techniques to display the spatial distribution of brain electrical activity. EEG topography and tomography are being used in the diagnosis and treatment of mental disorders.[45]

8.3.4   The Pacemaker: 1958

Rune Elmqvist (1906–1996) developed the first implantable pacemaker in 1958 (See an implantable pacemaker, Fig. 13.8 in page 197), working under the direction of Åke Senning, senior physician and cardiac surgeon at the Karolinska University Hospital, Stockholm, Sweden.

Elmqvist initially worked as a medical doctor but later worked as an engineer and inventor.[46]

8.3.5   Hip Replacement: 1962

John Charnley (1911–1982) was an English orthopedic surgeon, innovator, and bio-engineer, recognized as the founder of modern hip replacement (total hip arthroplasty), in 1962.[47]

8.3.6   In Vitro Fertilization: 1959

Min Chueh Chang (1908–1991) was a Chinese American reproductive biologist. His specific area of study was the fertilization process in mammalian reproduction. Though his career produced findings that are important and valuable to many areas in the field of fertilization, including his work on in vitro fertilization, which led to the first test-tube baby in 1959, he was best known to the world for his contribution to the development of the combined oral contraceptive pill at the Worcester Foundation for Experimental Biology. This was the first combined oral contraceptive approved by the FDA in 1960.[48]

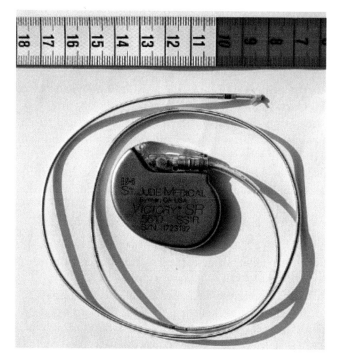

Figure 8.2   An implantable modern pacemaker. (https://en.wikipedia.org/wiki/ Artificial cardiac pacemaker)

8.3.7   First Polio Vaccine: 1956

Hilary Koprowski (1916–2013) was a Polish virologist and immunologist active in the United States, who demonstrated the world's first effective live polio vaccine.[49]

8.3.7.1   First Oral Polio Vaccine

Albert Sabin developed the first oral polio vaccine. The vaccine was tested on 100 million individuals between 1955 and 1961 and released in 1962.[50]

8.3.8   Cardiopulmonary Resuscitation: 1960

Peter J. Safar (1924–2003) was an Austrian physician, innovator, educator, and pioneer of cardiopulmonary resuscitation and critical care medicine.[51]

8.3.9   Beta-Blocker: 1962

Sir James Whyte Black (1924–2010) was a Scottish physician and pharmacologist. Black established a Veterinary Physiology Department at the University of Glasgow, where he became interested in the effects of adrenaline on the human heart. He went to work for ICI Pharmaceuticals in 1958 and, while there, developed propranolol, a beta-blocker used for the treatment of heart disease, in 1962. James Black was awarded the Nobel Prize in Physiology or Medicine in 1988 for the work leading to the development of propranolol and cimetidine. Cimetidine is a histamine H_2 receptor antagonist that inhibits stomach acid production. It is mainly used in the treatment of heartburn and peptic ulcers.[52]

8.3.10   Artificial Heart: 1963

Paul Winchell invented an artificial heart with the assistance of Henry Heimlich (the inventor of the Heimlich maneuver used to treat upper-airway obstructions, or choking, by foreign objects) and held the first patent for such a device. The University of Utah developed a similar apparatus around the same time, but when they tried to patent it, Winchell's heart was cited as prior art. The university requested that Winchell donate the heart to the University of Utah, which he did.[53]

8.3.11   First Liver Transplant: 1963

Thomas Earl Starzl (1926–2017) was an American physician, researcher, and expert on organ transplants. He performed the first human liver transplant and has often been referred to as the father of modern transplantation.[54]

8.3.12   First Lung Transplant: 1963

James D. Hardy (1918–2003) was a United States surgeon who performed the world's first human lung transplant.[55]

8.3.13   Valium (Diazepam): 1963

Leo Sternbach (May 1908–2005) was a Polish American chemist who is credited with first synthesizing benzodiazepines, the main class of tranquilizers, which refers to a drug that is designed for the treatment of anxiety, fear, tension, agitation, and disturbances of the mind, specifically to reduce states of anxiety and tension.[56]

8.3.14   First Vaccine for Measles: 1964

Maurice Ralph Hilleman (1919–2005) was a leading American microbiologist who specialized in vaccinology and developed over 40 vaccines, an unparalleled record of productivity. According to one estimate, his vaccines save nearly 8 million lives each year. Many have described him as one of the most influential vaccine developer of all time.[57]

8.3.15   First Portable Defibrillator: 1965

James Francis "Frank" Pantridge (1916–2004) was a Northern Irish physician, cardiologist, and professor who transformed emergency medicine and
paramedic services with the invention of the portable defibrillator.[58]

8.3.16   First Commercial Ultrasound: 1965

John Julian Cuttance Wild (1914–2009) was an English-born American physician who was part of the first group to use ultrasound for body imaging,
most notably for diagnosing cancer.[59]

8.3.17   First Human Pancreas Transplant: 1966

The first vascularized *pancreas* transplant was performed by William Kelly
and Richard Lillehei to treat a type 1 diabetes patient, in December 1966.
In December 1966, the first pancreas transplant ever was performed at the
University of Minnesota. R. Lillehei and W. Kelly transplanted a kidney and
a pancreas in a diabetic patient on dialysis, getting both organs functional.[60]

8.3.18   Rubella Vaccine: 1966

Dr. Harry Martin Meyer Jr. (1928–2001) directed the effort, with Dr. Paul D.
Parkman (1932–). Working rapidly, they introduced the first rubella vaccine
in 1966, assuring safe and lasting immunity at a low cost. Harry Martin Meyer
and Paul Parkman also devised a test to measure a person's immunity to
rubella.[61]

8.3.19   First Vaccine for Mumps: 1967

Maurice R. Hilleman (1919–2005) was a leading American microbiologist
who specialized in vaccinology and developed over 40 vaccines. (See earlier
note for more details.)[62]

8.3.20   First Human Heart Transplant: 1967

Christiaan Neethling Barnard (1922–2001) was a South African cardiac surgeon who performed the world's first human-to-human heart transplant
operation. On December 3, 1967, Barnard transplanted the heart of an accident victim Denise Darwall into the chest of 54-year-old Louis Washkansky,
with Washkansky regaining full consciousness and being able to talk easily
with his wife before dying 18 days later of pneumonia, largely brought on by
the anti-rejection drugs that suppressed his immune system.[63]

8.3.21   Powered Prothesis: 1968

Samuel W. Alderson (1914–2005) was an American inventor best known for
his development of the crash test dummy, a device that, during the last half

of the 20th century, was widely used by automobile manufacturers to test the reliability of automobile seat belts and other safety protocols. Samuel Alderson also made a strong contribution to healthcare through his development of the powered prosthesis.[64]

8.3.22   Controlled Drug Delivery: 1968

Alejandro Zaffaroni (1923–2014) was a serial entrepreneur who was responsible for founding several biotechnology companies in Silicon Valley. Products that he was involved in developing include the birth control pill, the nicotine patch, corticosteroids, and the DNA microarray.[65]

8.3.23   Balloon Catheter: 1969

Dr. Thomas J. "Tom" Fogarty (1934–) is an American surgeon and medical device inventor. He is best known for the invention of the embolectomy catheter (balloon catheter), which revolutionized the treatment of blood clots (embolus).[66]

8.3.24   Cochlear Implant: 1969

William F. House (1923–2012) was an American otologist, physician, and medical researcher who developed and invented the cochlear implant. The cochlear implant is the first invention to restore not just the sense of hearing but any of the absent five senses in humans. Dr. House also pioneered approaches to the lateral skull base for removal of tumors and is considered the father of neurotology.[67]

8.3.25   Cyclosporine, the First Effective Immunosuppressive Drug, Is Introduced in Organ Transplant Practice: 1970

Jean-François Borel (1933–) is a Belgian microbiologist and immunologist who is considered one of the discoverers of cyclosporin (immunosuppressant medication).[68]

8.3.26   MMR Vaccine: 1971

Maurice R. Hilleman (1919–2005) was a leading American microbiologist who specialized in vaccinology. (See earlier note for more details.)[69]

8.3.27   Genetically Modified Organisms: 1971

Ananda Mohan Chakrabarty, PhD (1938–2020), was an Indian American microbiologist, scientist, and researcher, most notable for his work in directed evolution and his role in developing a genetically engineered organism using plasmid transfer while working at General Electric. The patent for which led to the landmark Supreme Court case *Diamond v. Chakrabarty*. The result was that it became possible to patent new genetically modified organisms.[70]

8.3.28   First Commercial CT Scanner: 1971

Sir Godfrey Newbold Hounsfield (1919–2004) was an English electrical engineer who shared the 1979 Nobel Prize in Physiology or Medicine with Alan MacLeod Cormack for his part in developing the diagnostic technique of X-ray computed tomography (CT) or computerized tomography.

His name is immortalized in the Hounsfield scale, a quantitative measure of radiodensity used in evaluating CT scans. The scale is defined in Hounsfield units (symbol HU): running through the air, at –1000 HU; through water, at 0 HU; and up to the dense cortical bone, at +1000 HU and more.[71, 72]

8.3.29   Transdermal Patches: 1971

Alejandro Zaffaroni (1923–2014) was a biochemist in Uruguay with Italian descent.

Transdermal patches are patches that adhere to the skin to deliver drugs by being absorbed through the skin and into the bloodstream.[73]

8.3.30   Magnetic Resonance Imaging: 1971

Raymond Vahan Damadian (1936–) is an American physician of Armenian descent, medical practitioner, and inventor of the first MR (magnetic resonance) scanning machine.[74]

8.3.31   Insulin Pump: 1972

Dean Lawrence Kamen (1951–) is an American engineer, inventor, and businessman. He is known for inventing the Segway and iBOT, a powered wheelchair, as well as founding the nonprofit organization FIRST. Kamen holds over 1,000 patents.[75]

Personal Anecdote: The WWW Will Never Work!

During my first year at CERN, in 1972, I was there as a summer student, and every morning, all summer students from all over Europe and America had the privilege to go to the auditorium and listen to some very inspiring lectures. These lectures were mostly around particle physics and were very interesting. One morning, the lecture was about the World Wide Web. None of us had heard about this before. The lecture was about a new tool with the potential for collaboration and new findings for all particle physicists around the world. All are connected to this new technology platform, with the potential to speed up the developments inside particle physics.

Afterward, all summer students normally gathered for a quick coffee break before we went off to our respective departments.

The general comment during the coffee break from most of us was, "It will never work." We all know today how wrong we were in the summer of 1972.

We have all learned our lesson since then!

8.3.32   Laser Eye Surgery: 1973

Mani La Bhaumik (1931–) is an Indian American physicist and a bestselling author.

Bhaumik became the first student to receive a PhD degree from the Indian Institute of Technology Kharagpur, when he received his PhD in quantum physics in 1958. His thesis was on resonant electronic energy transfers, a subject very important for his work with lasers. His contributions to the development of new and high-power lasers merited his election by his peers to be a fellow of both the American Physical Society and the Institute of Electrical and Electronics Engineers.[76]

8.3.33   Development of the PET Scanner: 1973

Edward J. Hoffman (1942–2004), Michael E. Phelps (1939–), and Michael M. Ter-Pogossian (1925–1996) invented the positron-emission tomography (PET) scanner, which helps detect cancer, heart disease, and other serious illnesses.[77]

8.3.34   Liposuction (Cosmetic Surgery): 1974

Giorgio Fischer (19??—) is an Italian surgeon that spent most of his career in cosmetic surgery. The medical invention had importance for some people with extreme weight problems, but the very dominating application of the technique is cosmetic surgery. Dr. Giorgio Fischer and his son Dr. Giorgio Fischer Jr. did the first liposuction surgery.[78]

8.3.35   First Commercial PET Scanner

In 1961, James Robertson and his associates at Brookhaven National Laboratory built the first single-plane PET scan, nicknamed the head-shrinker. One of the factors most responsible for the acceptance of positron imaging was the development of radiopharmaceuticals.[79]

8.3.36   Last Fatal Case of Smallpox: 1978

In the summer of 1978, the last known case of smallpox was reported, claiming the life of 40-year-old medical photographer Janet Parker. How she got the disease was for a long time a mystery, but it was finally concluded that the virus came from a lab within the Birmingham Hospital where Janet Parker worked. The last natural case of which anywhere in the world had been reported in Somalia in 1977.[80]

8.3.37   Antiviral Drugs: 1979

Gertrude Belle Elion (1918–1999) and George H Hitchings (1905–1998) shared the Nobel Prize in Physiology or Medicine in 1988.

They were both American citizens and worked in the field of drug development and specifically in antiviral drugs. Both were biochemists and worked together for approximately half a century in drug development. Hitchings and Elion synthesized two antimetabolites, diaminopurine and thioguanine. This latter discovery led to a new drug, azathioprine, and a new application, organ transplants. Azathioprine suppressed the immune system, which would otherwise reject newly transplanted organs. In the 1960s, Hitchings and Elion determined that infectious diseases could be fought if drugs could be targeted to attack bacterial and viral DNA.[81]

8.3.38   First Commercial MRI Scanner: 1980

Raymond Damadian created the first MRI full-body scanner, which he nicknamed the Indomitable (unbeatable).[82]

8.3.39   Lithotripter: 1980

The German company Dornier launched the first lithotripter, which is a device using shock waves in order to destroy kidney and urinary stones noninvasively. The procedure is guided with the support of an X-ray or ultrasound.

The stones are smashed into small pieces, which makes them possible to be passed the normal way without pain.[83]

8.3.40   First Vaccine for Hepatitis B: 1980

The hepatitis B vaccine is a vaccine that prevents hepatitis B. The first dose is recommended within 24 hours of birth, with either two or three more doses given after that. This includes those with poor immune function, such as HIV/AIDS patients, and those born prematurely. It is also recommended that healthcare workers be vaccinated. In healthy people, routine immunization results in more than 95% of people being protected. The hepatitis B vaccine was developed by the American physician Baruch Blumberg. Blumberg won the Nobel Prize in Physiology or Medicine for his work on hepatitis B. The prize was shared with Daniel Carleton Gajdusek.[84]

8.3.41   Cloning of Interferons: 1980

Sydney Pestka (1936–2016) was an American biochemist and geneticist. Pestka was part of the team working on research involving the genetic code, protein synthesis, and ribosome function that led to the 1968 Nobel Prize in Physiology or Medicine received by Marshall Warren Nirenbery.

Interferons (IFNs) are proteins made and released by host cells in response to the presence of pathogens, such as viruses, bacteria, parasites, or tumor cells. They allow for communication among cells to trigger the protective defenses of the immune system that eradicate pathogens or tumors.[85]

8.3.42   Artificial Skin: 1981

John F. Burke (1922–2011) was an American medical researcher at Harvard University, widely known for his co-invention of synthetic skin in 1981, together with Dr. Ioannis V. Yannas (1935–), a physical chemist and engineer.

Artificial skin is a collagen scaffold that induces the regeneration of the skin in mammals, such as humans. The term was used in the late 1970s and early 1980s to describe a new treatment for massive burns.[86]

8.3.43   The First Human Heart-Lung Combined Transplant: 1981

The first heart-lung transplantation was performed in Houston by D.A. Cooley in 1968. Even though the girl who received this transplant survived only for 14 hours, this case showed that this kind of procedure can work. The first long-term survival was achieved by Bruce Reitz in 1981, at Stanford.[87]

8.3.44   Human Synthetic Insulin: 1982

Human insulin is the name that describes synthetic insulin, which is laboratory-grown to mimic insulin in humans. Human insulin was developed in the 1960s and 1970s and approved for pharmaceutical use in 1982. Eli Lilly was the first pharmaceutical company to produce human insulin.[88]

8.3.45   Automated DNA Sequencer: 1985

In 1986, Leroy Hood and Lloyd Smith from the California Institute of Technology developed the first semi-automatic DNA sequencer, working with a laser that recognized fluorescent DNA markers.[89]

8.3.46   Polymerase Chain Reaction: 1985

Kary Mullis (1944–2019) was an American biochemist. In recognition of his role in the invention of the polymerase chain reaction (PCR) technique. He shared the 1993 Nobel Prize in Chemistry with Michael Smith. PCR became a central technique in biochemistry and molecular biology and biochemistry.

PCR is a method widely used to rapidly develop millions to billions of copies (complete copies or partial copies) of a specific DNA sample, allowing scientists to take a very small sample of DNA and amplify it (or a part of it) to a large enough amount to study in detail.[90]

8.3.47   Surgical Robot: 1985

Dr. Yik San Kwoh is the inventor of the robot, the software interface program used in the first robot-aided surgery.[91]

8.3.48   DNA Fingerprinting: 1985

Alec Jeffreys (1950–) is a British geneticist that developed techniques for genetic fingerprinting and DNA profiling, which are now used worldwide in forensic science.[92]

8.3.49   Fluoxetine HCI: 1986

Fluoxetine was discovered by Eli Lilly and Company in 1972 and entered medical use in 1986. It is on the World Health Organization's List of Essential Medicines. It is available as a generic medication.

Note: A generic drug is a pharmaceutical drug that contains the same chemical substance as a drug that was originally protected by chemical patents. Generic drugs are allowed for sale after the patents on the original drugs expire. Because the active chemical substance is the same, the medical profile of generics is believed to be equivalent in performance.[93]

8.3.50   First Separation of Occipital Craniopagus Twins: 1987

Benjamin Carson (1951–), an American scientist, did a successful separation of occipital craniopagus twins in 1987 with a huge team of 70 persons. Carson used a radical approach, in which the twins' body temperatures were lowered to the point of circulatory arrest. The success of the procedure and the reconstructive techniques employed gained Carson world renown as a pediatric neurosurgeon. In 2012, he became a politician on the conservative side.[94]

8.3.51   Commercially Available Statins: 1987

The drug dramatically reduced cholesterol levels and was well tolerated. No tumors were detected. In November 1986, Merck sent the New Drug Application (NDA) to the FDA in the United States, and lovastatin was given FDA approval to become the first commercial statin in September 1987.

Approximately 30 million people have been treated with the drug.[95]

8.3.52   Tissue Engineering: 1987

Joseph Vacanti (1948–) and Robert Langer (1948–) are the two scientists that are behind the concept of tissue engineering. Vacanti is a pediatric surgeon and Langer is a biochemist. Tissue engineering is a rather new field of science, medicine, and engineering, in which living replacements for organs and tissues of the body are designed and built. Cells from a person can be taken out from a patient's organ and then grown in a lab and then incorporated back into the patient in order to heal a specific function or organ. The cells taken out are put into a type of scaffold consisting of a type of special plastic. The process is a type of organ building and/or renovation.

Regenerative medicine is more focused on using stem cell regenerative therapy to kick-start the patient's body's healing processes with their own stem cells, rather than utilizing lab-grown replacements and tissue scaffolds. This natural process is less about replacing non-functioning tissue by growing new cells and more about stimulating the body to replace them itself using stem cell therapy and stem cell treatments.

The goal of the two disciplines is rather similar, but the way they operate is rather different.[96]

8.3.53   Intravascular Stent: 1988

Julio Palmaz (1945–) is a doctor of vascular radiology at the University of Texas Health Science Center in San Antonio. Together with Dr. Richard Schatz, a cardiologist from Brooke Army Medical Center, developed the first intravascular stent, the Palmaz–Schatz stent, in 1988. A stent is a metal or plastic tube inserted into the lumen of an anatomic vessel or duct to keep the passageway open. With a special balloon catheter, the stent can be transported to the place in the vessel where it is aimed to expand the vessel and give free passage for the blood.

To further reduce the incidence of restenosis, the drug-eluting stent was introduced in 2003.[97]

8.3.54   Laser Cataract Surgery: 1988

Patricia Bath (1942–2019) was the first African American to complete a residency in ophthalmology in 1973.

Bath invented the laserphaco probe, improving treatment for cataract patients. She patented the device in 1988, becoming the first African American female doctor to receive a medical patent.[98]

8.3.55   Pre-Implementation Genetic Diagnosis: 1989

The aim of pre-implantation genetic diagnosis (PGD) is to characterize the genetic status of the cells (usually single cells) that have been biopsied from oocytes/zygotes or embryos created in vitro during assisted reproductive treatment. PGD is a multi-step procedure that requires close collaboration between gynecologists who are experts in assisted reproduction, embryologists who are experts in micromanipulation of germ cells, and in embryo biopsy and geneticists who are experts in genetic analysis at the single-cell level.[99]

8.3.56   DNA Microarray: 1989

Stephen Fodor (1953–) is a scientist and businessman in the field of DNA microarray technology. He is the founder of Affymetrix, a company that produces DNA microarrays to screen gene expression and genetic variations in large portions of genomes, such as from humans, rats, and mice, which is currently widely used in research and could be used to screen patients for diseases.[100]

8.3.57   Gamow Bag: 1990

Rustem Igor Gamow (1935–2021) is a former microbiology professor at the University of Colorado and an inventor. His best known inventions include the Gamow bag (it is primarily used for treating severe cases of altitude sickness, high-altitude cerebral edema, and high-altitude pulmonary edema) and the shallow underwater breathing apparatus (a device for breathing underwater for approximately 10 minutes).[101]

8.3.58   First Vaccine for Hepatitis A

The hepatitis A vaccine is a vaccine that prevents hepatitis type A.

It is effective in around 95% of cases and lasts for at least 20 years and possibly a person's entire life. If given, two doses are recommended beginning after the age of 1. It is given by injection into a muscle.

The first hepatitis A vaccine was approved in Europe in 1991 and in the United States in 1995. It is on the World Health Organization's List of Essential Medicines. There are three main types of hepatitis: hepatitis A, B, and C. Hepatitis C can be more severe and is the most lethal, but even those with acute illness can recover without lasting liver damage.[102]

8.3.59   Electroactive Polymers (Artificial Muscle): 1992

Electroactive polymers, or EAPs, are polymers that exhibit a change in size or shape when stimulated by an electric field. The most common applications of this type of material are in actuators and sensors. A typical characteristic property of an EAP is that it will undergo a large amount of deformation while sustaining large forces.[103]

8.3.60   Intracytoplasmic Sperm Injection: 1992

Paul Devroey and Andre van Steirteghem: Intracytoplasmic sperm injection (ICSI) is an assisted reproductive technology (ART) used to treat sperm-related infertility problems. ICSI is used to enhance the fertilization phase of in vitro fertilization (IVF) by injecting a single sperm into a mature egg.[104]

8.3.61   Adult Stem Cell Used in Regeneration of
Tissues and Organs In Vivo: 1995

Adult stem cells have been identified in most mammalian tissues of the adult body and are known to support the continuous repair and regeneration of tissues. A generalized decline in tissue regenerative responses associated with age is believed to result from a depletion and/or a loss of function of adult stem cells, which itself may be a driving cause of many age-related disease pathologies.[105]

8.3.62   Dolly the Sheep Cloned: 1996

Dolly (July 5, 1996–February 14, 2003) was a female Finnish Dorset sheep and the first cloned from an adult somatic cell. She was cloned by associates of the Roslin Institute in Scotland, using the process of nuclear transfer from a cell taken from a mammary gland. Her cloning proved that a cloned organism could be produced from a mature cell from a specific body part. Contrary to popular belief, she was not the first animal to be cloned.[106]

8.3.63   Stem Cell Therapy: 1998

James Alexander Thomson (1958–) is an American developmental biologist, best known for deriving the first human embryonic stem cell line in 1998 and for deriving human-induced pluripotent stem cells (iPS) in 2007.

The Thomson Lab was the first to report the successful isolation of human embryonic stem cells. On November 6, 1998, *Science* published this research in an article titled "Embryonic Stem Cell Lines Derived from Human Blastocysts," the results of which *Science* later featured in its "Scientific Breakthrough of the Year" article, in 1999.[107]

8.4   Summary of the Developments in the 20th Century

The hospital where I worked as a hospital physicist, Linköping University Hospital, was very advanced in medical technology development and built early collaboration with clinical specialties. A lot of experimental setups were ongoing in many different labs for testing ideas and measurements on patients. The collaboration among clinicians, physicists, and technologists was unique and rather early, as seen from a Nordic perspective.

They all had patient consent and ethical approval. Still, they were not always ready for clinical launch, and situations could look rather complicated. See the illustration in Figure 8.3.

The rapid progress of medicine in this era was reinforced by enormous improvements in communication among scientists throughout the world. Through publications, and later in the century, computers and electronic media, scientists and clinicians could freely exchange ideas and report on their results and outcomes. It became less common for scientists and

Medical technology introduced in clinical environment

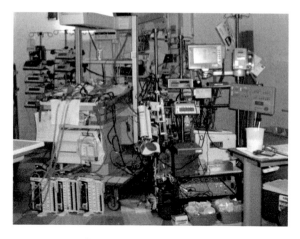

Where is the patient?

Figure 8.3   Very early clinical tests of some prototype cardiovascular measurements.
Maybe not so patient-friendly or medical staff–tested/proofed. (Photo by Bengt
Nielsen; from University Hospital in Linköping, Sweden; approximately 1982.)[108]

clinicians to work as individuals, as teamwork became more and more
prominent.

In the first half of the century, the focus continued to be on combating
infections, and landmarks were also attained in endocrinology, nutrition,
and other areas. In the years following World War II, insights came from cell
biology, which altered the basic concepts of the disease process. New discoveries in biochemistry and physiology opened the way for more precise diagnostic tests, and this gave more effective therapies. The spectacular advances
in biomedical engineering enabled physicians and surgeons to probe into
structures and functions of the human body by noninvasive techniques, such
as ultrasound (US), computerized tomography (CT), and magnetic resonance imaging (MRI). With each new scientific development, the medical
practices of just a few years earlier became rather obsolete.

Reference List, Chapter 8

1 www.nobelprize.org/prizes/medicine/1930/landsteiner/biographical/
2 https://en.wikipedia.org/wiki/Alzheimer%27s_disease
3 https://en.wikipedia.org/w/index.php?go=Go&search=Willem+Einthoven.&titl
   e=Special%3ASearch&ns0=1
4 www.nobelprize.org/prizes/medicine/1908/ehrlich/biographical/
5 https://pubmed.ncbi.nlm.nih.gov/8209988/
6 www.umassmed.edu/dcoe/diabetes-education/patient-resources/banting-and-best-
   discover-insulin/

7   https://en.wikipedia.org/wiki/Timeline_of_human_vaccines
8   www.sciencehistory.org/historical-profile/howard-walter-florey-and-ernst-boris-chain
9   www.ncbi.nlm.nih.gov/pmc/articles/PMC6351694/
10 https://en.wikipedia.org/wiki/Alexander_Fleming
11 www.nobelprize.org/prizes/medicine/1929/hopkins/biographical/
12 https://academic.oup.com/endo/article-abstract/129/5/2271/2535297?redirectedFrom=fulltext
13 https://pubmed.ncbi.nlm.nih.gov/8916353/
14 https://pubmed.ncbi.nlm.nih.gov/1093589/
15 www.nobelprize.org/prizes/medicine/1927/wagner-jauregg/facts/121; www.jstor.org/stable/48508231
16 https://pubmed.ncbi.nlm.nih.gov/20798415/
17 https://pubmed.ncbi.nlm.nih.gov/?term=https%3A%2F%2Fwww.neuroelectrics.com%2Fblog%2F2014%2F12%2F18%2Fhans-berger-lights-and-shadows-of-the-inventor-of-electroencephalography%2F
18 https://en.wikipedia.org/wiki/Christine_Jorgensen
19 https://en.wikipedia.org/wiki/Christiaan_Eijkman
20 www.britannica.com/biography/Manfred-J-Sakel
21 www.encyclopedia.com/science/encyclopedias-almanacs-transcripts-and-maps/julius-wagner-jauregg
22 www.nobelprize.org/prizes/medicine/1949/moniz/article/
23 www.ncbi.nlm.nih.gov/pmc/articles/PMC6469031/
24 https://pubmed.ncbi.nlm.nih.gov/11940939/
25 www.medicaldiscoverynews.com/shows/214_mammogramOrigins.html
26 www.nobelprize.org/prizes/physics/1936/anderson/facts/
27 https://history.aip.org/exhibits/lawrence/first.htm
28 https://healthimaging.com/topics/medical-imaging/diagnostic-imaging/ahra-2008/pet-scanner-innovator-gordon-l-brownell-dies
29 www.worldscientific.com/doi/10.1142/9789814289764_0010
30 www.sciencedirect.com/topics/nursing-and-health-professions/endotracheal-tube
31 https://case.edu/ech/articles/b/beck-claude-schaeffer
32 https://www.nobelprize.org/prizes/medicine/1970/axelrod/biographical/
33 www.nobelprize.org/prizes/medicine/1994/gilman/biographical/
34 https://pubmed.ncbi.nlm.nih.gov/11729731/
35 https://historycambridge.org/articles/the-remarkable-john-jack-emerson-founder-of-the-j-h-emerson-company-by-daphne-abeel/
36 www.sciencehistory.org/historical-profile/james-watson-francis-crick-maurice-wilkins-and-rosalind-franklin
37 www.jstor.org/stable/769894
38 https://pubmed.ncbi.nlm.nih.gov/15039985/
39 https://jdc.jefferson.edu/jeffhistoryposters/1/
40 www.historyofinformation.com/detail.php?entryid=1670
41 www.ncbi.nlm.nih.gov/pmc/articles/PMC6482420/
42 https://en.wikipedia.org/wiki/Vacuum_extraction
43 https://timenote.info/en/Lloyd-Conover
44 https://pubmed.ncbi.nlm.nih.gov/16455257/
45 https://en.wikipedia.org/wiki/Artificial cardiac pacemaker
46 https://en.wikipedia.org/wiki/John_Charnley

47 https://en.wikipedia.org/wiki/Min_Chueh_Chang; www.nobelprize.org/prizes/medicine/1988/black/biographical/

48 www.ncbi.nlm.nih.gov/pmc/articles/PMC3719820/

49 www.sabin.org/about/our-history/dr-albert-b-sabin/

50 https://en.wikipedia.org/wiki/Peter_Safar 136

51 https://en.wikipedia.org/wiki/James_Black_(pharmacologist)

52 https://leaps.org/artificial-heart-paul-winchell/a-meeting-of-the-minds

53 www.ncbi.nlm.nih.gov/pmc/articles/PMC8968477/

54 www.ncbi.nlm.nih.gov/pmc/articles/PMC5757055/

55 www.ncbi.nlm.nih.gov/pmc/articles/PMC8968477/

56 https://en.wikipedia.org/wiki/Maurice_Hilleman

57 https://https://en.wikipedia.org/wiki/Frank_Pantridge

58 www. https://en.wikipedia.org/wiki/John_J._Wild

59 https://https://pubmed.ncbi.nlm.nih.gov/28595751/

60 www/Dr-Harry-Martin-Meyer-vaccine-innovator-72–2882202.php

61 https://en.wikipedia.org/wiki/Maurice_Hilleman

62 https://https://en.wikipedia.org/wiki/Christiaan_Barnard

63 https://en.wikipedia.org/wiki/Samuel_W._Alderson

64 https://medium.com/lsf-magazine/alejandro-zaffaroni-3abae75e53ed

65 https://vascularnews.com/profile-tom-fogarty

66 https://https://en.wikipedia.org/wiki/William_F._House

67 https://https://en.wikipedia.org/wiki/Jean-Fran%C3%A7ois_Borel

68 www.ncbi.nlm.nih.gov/pmc/articles/PMC7150172/

69 https://https://en.wikipedia.org/wiki/Ananda_Mohan_Chakrabarty

70 www.google.com/search?client=safari&rls=en&q=Sir+Godfrey+Newbold+Hounsfield&ie=UTF-8&oe=UTF-8

71 www.google.com/search?client=safari&rls=en&q=Sir+Godfrey+Newbold+Hounsfield&ie=UTF-8&oe=UTF-8

72 www.tapemark.com/blog/transdermal-patches

73 www.invent.org/inductees/alejandro-zaffaroni

74 https://https://en.wikipedia.org/wiki/Raymond_Damadian

75 www.multi-mania.be/dean-kamen/

76 https://bhaumik-institute.physics.ucla.edu/biography

77 www.ncbi.nlm.nih.gov/pmc/articles/PMC5374360/

78 www.ncbi.nlm.nih.gov/pmc/articles/PMC2825130/

79 https://https://web.eng.fiu.edu/godavart/bme4531-sp12/PET_Student_ppt-Spring2012.pdf

80 www.cdc.gov/smallpox/history/history.html

81 www.nobelprize.org/womenwhochangedscience/stories/gertrude-elion

82 www.nytimes.com/2022/08/17/science/raymond-damadian-dead.html

83 www.dornier.com/important-day-medical-history/

84 www.cdc.gov/mmwr/preview/mmwrhtml/mm5125a3.htm

85 www.sciencedirect.com/science/article/abs/pii/S1359610107000780

86 https://en.wikipedia.org/wiki/John_F._Burke

87 https://125.stanford.edu/first-heart-lung-transplant/

88 https://diabetes.org/blog/history-wonderful-thing-we-call-insulin

89 www.sciencedirect.com/science/article/abs/pii/0888754387900462

90 www.nobelprize.org/prizes/chemistry/1993/mullis/facts/

91 www.edubilla.com/invention/surgical-robot/

92 https://embryo.asu.edu/pages/alec-john-jeffreys-1950

93   www.ncbi.nlm.nih.gov/pmc/articles/PMC3894728/
94   http://en.wikipedia.org/wiki/Patrick_and_Benjamin_Binder
95   www.ncbi.nlm.nih.gov/pmc/articles/PMC3108295/
96   https://langer-lab.mit.edu/sites/default/files/documents/Science-1993-Langer-920-6.pdf
97   www.invent.org/inductees/julio-c-palmaz
98   www.invent.org/inductees/patricia-bath
99   https://pubmed.ncbi.nlm.nih.gov/19793305/
100 https://dnalc.cshl.edu/view/16757-Biography-36-Stephen-P-A-Fodor-1953-.html
101 https://en.wikipedia.org/wiki/Igor_Gamow
102 www.ncbi.nlm.nih.gov/pmc/articles/PMC6823267/
103 https://link.springer.com/book/10.1007/978-1-84628-372-7
104 https://en.wikipedia.org/wiki/Paul_Devroey
105 www.ncbi.nlm.nih.gov/pmc/articles/PMC2475560/
106 www.britannica.com/topic/Dolly-cloned-sheep
107 https://en.wikipedia.org/wiki/James_Thomson_(cell_biologist)
108 Photo of experimental MedTech lab at Linköping University Hospital, approximately 1982, photo taken by Bengt Nielsen.

Chapter 9

MODERN MEDICINE: FROM DIAGNOSIS TO THERAPY

9.1 Modern Imaging Techniques

9.1.1 Let's Go a Bit Deeper into the Different Imaging Techniques

All imaging techniques developed are using some type of electromagnetic radiation, and this is why an in-depth understanding of light was so important. In Figure 9.1, you can see the different wavelengths and the frequencies they use. The ionizing techniques are to the left with the highest frequencies, and these imaging modalities can cause biological hazards. The lowest frequencies are to the right, and these imaging modalities are the ones that we know as the safe ones.

9.1.1.1 Radiology

Radiography led to the development of radiology and also to the development of modern medicine. In addition, it led to the exponential development of today's many new imaging techniques built around other and new phenomena and principles. Today, we count on these techniques or modalities as obligatory diagnostic efforts, and they have become a commodity for

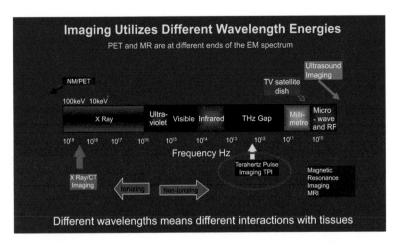

Figure 9.1 Definitions of wavelengths and frequencies for the different imaging techniques. (Illustration created by Bengt Nielsen.)[1]

DOI: 10.1201/9781003393320-11

almost every possible disease diagnosis. The many imaging techniques introduced after the introduction of radiography are, in most parts of the world, gathered under the radiology service within our healthcare system.

9.1.1.2   The Principles and Techniques in the Early Days of Radiology

The introduction of routine X-ray diagnostics reached the whole world more or less instantaneously. During the first 60–70 years of the 20th century, X-ray techniques were enhanced and adapted to be used in the majority of clinical situations at hospitals and clinics around the world. Let's look at the technological developments we have been witnessing through the years since the introduction of X-ray diagnostics.

9.1.2   Different X-ray Tubes

See Figures 9.2, 9.3, and 9.4.

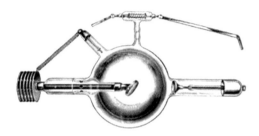

Figure 9.2   Cathode-ray tube/Crookes tube, around 1910. (https://commons. wikimedia.org/w/index.php?curid=1433630)[2]

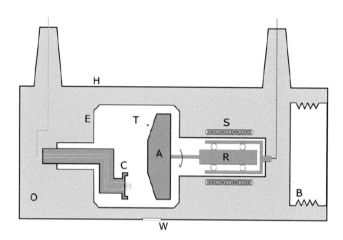

Figure 9.3   Simplified rotating anode tube schematic. A, anode; C, cathode; T, anode target; and W, X-ray window. (ChumpusRex. http://en.wikipedia.org/wiki/ Image: X-ray tube in housing.png, CC BY-SA 3.0)[3]

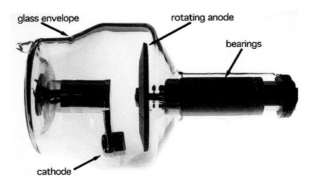

Figure 9.4   Modern X-ray tube with a rotating anode. (en.wikipedia.org)[4]

9.1.3   The Principle of X-rays Made Simple

The very early X-ray tubes, the Coolidge and Crookes tubes, have both residual gases in the tube, and the generation of X-rays was through ionization when a high voltage (50,000–150,000 volts) is applied between the cathode and the anode.

Modern X-ray tubes instead have a high level of vacuum inside the tube, and the electrons are produced by having a filament, a small circuit that is heated through a current and leads to the freed electrons will be dragged to the anode where the X-rays are generated. The biggest challenge in making the X-ray tube is the heating of the anode when electrons from the filament hit the anode. This is the reason why modern X-ray tubes have anodes made of tungsten and rotating anodes that distribute the heat over a larger area. It complicates the construction of the X-ray tube, as before exposure, the rotating anode must be accelerated to 3,000–4,000 rotations per minute before exposure.

The dominating factor when designing an X-ray tube is that the anode needs to be able to tolerate very high temperatures. Tungsten, with a melting temperature of 3,370°C, is, therefore, today still the material of choice for the anode.

The X-ray beam is directed toward the organ of the patient to be imaged, and a diaphragm is used on the X-ray tube in order to irradiate a volume as small as possible. First, because we want to give the patient a low radiation dose and, second, because scattered radiation is generated in the patient that gives rise to degradation of the image quality.

The X-ray spectrum shows the intensity of different photon energies coming out of the X-ray tube. The different energies arise when the accelerated electrons are penetrating the anode, and the X-ray photons are created. The lower energies will not penetrate through the body part you will image and will consequently only give radiation to the patient. Therefore, these energies are filtered directly at the output from the X-ray tube by the addition of different metallic filters, like aluminum or copper. The two sharp peaks that are seen in the spectrum in Figure 9.5 are an effect of what

The X-ray spectrum – output from the X-ray tube

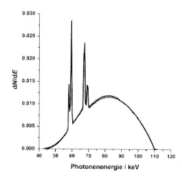

Figure 9.5   The X-ray spectrum, tube voltage is 110 kV. (Bengt Nielsen, Thesis 1985, Linköping University, Sweden.)[5]

is called characteristic X-rays. Characteristic X-rays are emitted when outer-shell electrons fill a vacancy in the inner shell of an atom, releasing X-rays in a pattern that is characteristic of each element. Characteristic X-rays were discovered by Charles Glover Barka in 1909, who later won the Nobel Prize in Physics in 1917 for his discovery.

9.1.4   High-Voltage Generator

X-ray units require a high-voltage generator to achieve the necessary power required by an X-ray tube. AC power will supply X-ray units with sinusoidal currents, resulting in peaks and troughs, limiting an X-ray tube to produce X-rays only half of the 1/60th-of-a-second cycle.

A single-phase high-voltage generator converts this AC power into a half- or full-wave rectified supply with a measure in the thousands of volts.

The half-wave rectification results in a peak voltage that will dip to zero, reoccurring; this will consequently influence the behavior of radiation produced, and hence, the name *kilovoltage peak* (kVp) was born. The advancement of high-voltage generators from single-phase to three-phase to constant potential generators has overcome this voltage ripple, creating a continuous, uninterrupted voltage. Modern X-ray units, which largely utilize constant potential generators, do not have voltage ripple and, consequently, employ the term *kV* (kilovoltage) rather than *kVp* (kilovoltage peak).

When we learned how to protect ourselves from X-rays, we also had to learn how to handle the risks of the early days of open, high tension in X-ray rooms (Figure 9.6).

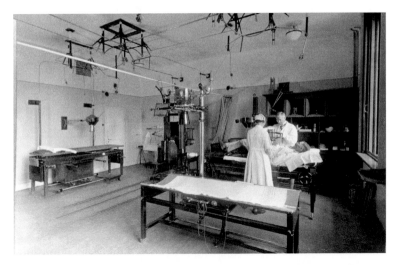

Figure 9.6   The Roentgen Institute in Lund, Sweden, around 1918. Note the different types of patient beds and the open high-tension cables in the ceiling. (With courtesy of Medical Collections of Region Skåne, Sweden. Photographer: Per Bagge.)[6]

9.1.5   Detection of X-ray Images

When the X-rays passed through the patient's body to be imaged, the latent image was registered by some type of media in order to be reviewed by a radiologist (Figure 9.7). The X-ray, in the early days of X-rays, was registered directly on a film with a rather thick silver emulsion after the X-rays had passed the patient. At the beginning of the X-ray era, the radiation burden on the patient was heavy, and new inventions were rapidly developed.

By inserting a registering film in between a pair of fluorescent screens and, hereby, letting the film emulsion be exposed to the fluorescent light instead of by direct X-rays, the radiation dose could be reduced by up to 100 times.

The X-rays interacted with the fluorescent screen, and the fluorescent material lit up and exposed the film. When fluoroscopy was done, meaning registration of the patient's body directly by the radiologist, the light from the screen was so faint that it had to be very dark in the room in order to see anything. At the beginning of the era of Roentgen, it was a discipline mainly in the dark. All these challenges were resolved as X-ray technology developed during the following decade at the start of the 20th century.

When Roentgen recorded the first images of the hand of his wife, Bertha, he used sensitized glass photographic plates. Soon, the glass plates were replaced by photographic films with a silver-based emulsion.

The glass plates were unpractical to handle when large volumes of X-rays started to become common. The expansion of the use of medical X-rays was

Detection of the X-rays behind the patient – image-registration

Direct film need to have a thick silver emulsion:
Resulting in high radiation dose to the patient.

X-ray cassett – fluorescence light will expose the film:
Medium radiation dose .

Figure 9.7   Different methods to register the X-ray image before there were direct digital X-ray solutions. (Bengt Nielsen, Thesis 1985, Linköping University, Sweden.)[7]

extremely fast, and many new technology developments making the use of Roentgen more and more practical entered the market very rapidly.

In the very early days of fluoroscopy (dynamic examinations) when the radiologist was observing the patient's organs behind the fluorescent screen, it was realized that the radiologist was hit with all the penetrating X-rays coming through the fluorescent screen. It became obvious that the radiologist had to be protected. The solution was to insert a glass screen between the fluorescent screen and the radiologist. The glass window was made of lead-doped glass (lead glass).

These types of exams were rather challenging, as the very faint image on the fluorescent screen demanded complete darkness in the X-ray room, and the radiologist needed to be darkness-adopted before entering the examination room.

Very quickly, the need for documented images led to the development of the X-ray film. When X-ray film was introduced, it led to the option for the radiologist to review the pictures after the X-ray image had been taken and read/diagnosed on a lightbox. Hereby, the images and cases could then be discussed with other radiologists and physicians.

The latent image (the invisible image that bears the information of the X-rays having passed the human object being X-rayed) was detected on a photographic film with a silver emulsion. As the X-ray photons are very energetic, only a small fraction of the X-rays is detected. The direct film emulsion had to be rather thick in order to capture a fraction of the photons coming from the passage of the patient.

Direct X-ray films were used for high-resolution skeleton imaging until the early 1970s. Already during the 1960s, we learned how to reduce the radiation dose by putting light-sensitive film between two fluorescent screens in a cassette. The X-rays produced fluorescent light when they hit the screens, and this light exposed the film. By this arrangement, the resolution was slightly diminished, but the radiation dose to the patient was reduced substantially.

The exposed cassettes were transported to a darkroom for development. The cassettes were, thereafter, reloaded with new film and used for the next X-ray exam.

9.2   The Conventional X-ray Image

The X-ray image is a projection of a three-dimensional body part that is projected onto a two-dimensional image. This makes the X-ray images rather complicated to interpret. Those parts of the body that are close to the X-ray tube will become magnified more than the parts of the body that are closer to the detector.

The radiologists became very skilled in interpreting the images, and a lot of this skill was that they knew the body anatomy very well. Clinicians who asked for an X-ray most of the time needed help in interpreting the resulting images. When you take a conventional X-ray, everything that you will see on the film is a projection of the trajectories of the X-rays as they pass through the body. This means that the things that are closer to the X-ray tube will be magnified more, and the structures that are closer to the detector/film will be less magnified.

If you want to have a sharp image of a certain detail/structure in the body, you need to do a tomography (Figure 9.8). This means that everything that is either above or below a tomographic plan will be blurred, while the structures within the slice will be sharp. The blurring is the consequence of the movement of the X-ray tube and the detector/film while doing the exposure.

The tomography method was a very common radiology procedure until the invention of computerized tomography (CT) was introduced in the late 1970s.

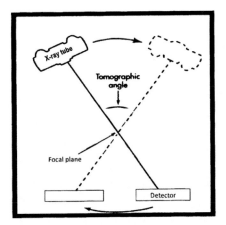

Figure 9.8   The principle of X-ray tomography. (Bengt Nielsen, made for my dissertation lecture.)[8]

Today, it is hard to think of any situation when you would prefer conventional tomography. The only reason would be if you do not have access to a CT. The CT can accomplish what sometimes is called the ideal tomography compared to the conventional technique.

With a normal projection, it would have been impossible to see the small bones inside our ears. By moving the X-ray tube simultaneously with the detector/film cassette during the exposure time, a single plane will be imaged sharply, and the planes above and below the chosen plane will be blurred. This procedure is called tomography.

Around 1985, direct digital detectors were introduced in most Radiology Departments, and film development machines were gradually expelled.

The introduction was stepwise, and many departments did it in two steps. Step 1 was what was called computerized radiology (CR), and the latent image was detected on a screen in the X-ray room inside a type of cassette and then taken to a reader where the image could be visualized. Gradually, this has been replaced by direct digital equipment adapted to each specific clinical exam. The detectors used are pixel-based with materials that convert the X-ray interaction very effectively with very low radiation doses.

The CR systems are still available for many mobile applications outside the Radiology Department; for instance, bedside lung CRs.

During the days I worked as a hospital physicist in a Radiology Department at the beginning of the 1970s, we did many dynamic contrast studies with frame rates of around 2–10 images per second, with film changers synchronized with contrast injections in order to study blood flow in the legs, brain, and in fact, every part of the body where studies of blood flow were needed. These analog film studies were technically cumbersome compared to the technique available today but served their purpose well in those days.

During the 1970s and 1980s, we also performed a lot of dynamic contrast studies of the heart by filming the heart and its vessels at a very high rate to capture images of the beating heart. The filming cameras were very similar to what the film industry used. The image came from an X-ray image intensifier (see Figure 9.9).

An image intensifier is a full-size vacuum tube covering the patient's body, and the output screen is small enough so that a film camera could image it. Through the large minification in the image intensifier, the image that the TV camera tube is looking at is very intense/bright and, hence, produces excellent image quality. See the principle in Figure 9.9.

Fluoroscopic techniques (real-time imaging and dynamic exams) are used for live exams when you would like to study blood flow in different parts of the body, study the stomach function by injection of contrast media, and dynamically study the contrast media transport through the digestive system, or simply position a certain body part for an ordinary X-ray image.

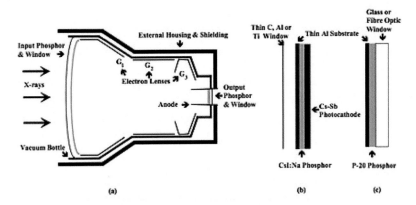

Figure 9.9   The principle of the buildup of an image intensifier tube, including a TV camera tube. (en.wikipedia.org/wiki)[9]

Normally, fluoroscopic imaging is obtained through the introduction of contrast media. For X-rays, the contrast media used is iodine, or for stomach studies, barium is used. The original technique is shown in Figure 9.9.

The image intensifier is a vacuum tube with the frontal phosphor (input screen) toward the patient receiving the X-ray photons, coming from the patient after passing through the patient's body. The input phosphor screen made of cesium iodide (CsI) converts the latent image into an electron pattern that is focused down to a size of approximately 20 mm. The focusing is done by some focusing lenses, and at the same time, there is an accelerating electric field applied between the input and the output screen. The minification will render a very strong illuminated screen that a TV camera will be looking at. The output screen in the image intensifier will convert the electrons into visible light made of silver-activated zinc cadmium sulfide (ZnCdS:Ag). The screen image is then sent to a TV monitor for the radiologist to look at. X-ray image intensifiers were very expensive, and they did not last for very long either. Each time they were replaced, it cost US$7,000 to US$12,000, depending on the size of the intensifier tube. The average lifetime was depending on the use, but more than 5 years' lifetime was unusual.

It was a rather bulky technique at the time of introduction, but these fluoroscopic X-ray suites were very common all over the world from the late 1950s. At the time, being a hospital physicist from 1978 to 1987, we had four X-ray rooms of this kind in a department with 20 X-ray rooms.

Today, most of the image intensifiers have been replaced with full-size direct digital imaging plates. It is cheaper and much less bulky. Moreover, it had an improved image quality and lower radiation dose, both to the patient and to the X-ray personnel.

9.3   Angiography

Angiography is a medical imaging technique used to visualize the inside, or lumen, of blood vessels and organs of the body, with particular interest on the arteries, veins, and heart chambers. This is traditionally done by injecting a radio-opaque contrast agent, like iodine, into the blood vessel. See Figure 9.10. In Figure 9.11 a simlar imaging technique is used but now obtained with CT. The visualization of a coronary veseel (in the heart). Note the clearly visual calcifications in the coronary vessel.

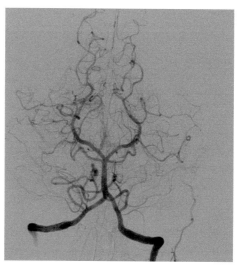

Figure 9.10   Angiogram, frontal view of the brain. Cerebral angiography, left vertebra injection. (en.wikipedia.org)[10]

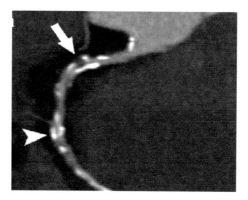

Figure 9.11   Image of contrast-enhanced dual-source CT angiograph. Accuracy of angiography: First experience in a coronary population without heart rate; dual-source CT, high pre-test probability. (commons.wikimedia.org)[11]

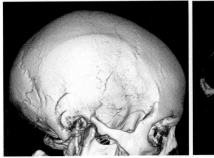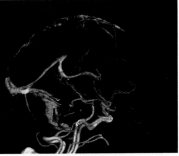

Figure 9.12 Volume-rendered venous-phase CT angiography of the head of a 41-year-old woman who had cerebral sinus thrombosis on previous CT angiographies but no abnormality this time. Both images are from the same scan, but the image on the right uses automatic bone removal, as well as the removal of some extra-cranial vessels. (Mikael Hällström, commons.wikimedia.org)[12]

In Figure 9.12, a CT angiography is shown where the same scan is used to reconstruct both the skull image of the head as well as the blood vessels. As the images are digital several images of different CT values can be reconstructed.

Dynamic imaging used X-ray-based techniques, such as fluoroscopy or the earlier used film-changer techniques, where pictures are taken at different time intervals in order to diagnose things like stroke, cerebral bleedings, aneurysms (an aneurysm is an outward bulging, likened to a bubble or balloon, caused by a localized, abnormal, weak spot on a blood vessel), or other vascular diseases where it is necessary/mandatory to do angiographies.

The drawback is that such an exam is a slightly invasive exam, as contrast needs to be inserted into an artery or a vein. Hence, the exam had to be done in a sterile environment. In addition, the exam also carried some risks for the patient. Angiograms need a contrast injection with iodine and can be done in many parts of the body when you want to see the local or specific blood flow in the heart, in the legs, in the kidney, and so on.

Computerized Tomography (CT): The first imaging technique linked with a computer in order to reconstruct (calculate) the final image (Figure 9.13 and Figure 9.14a).

This was a breakthrough for clinical imaging to become not only digital but also quantitative.

The possibilities of X-ray technology were further expanded with CT. If X-rays are sent through the body from different angles and registered when they have passed the body, images of different cross-sections are created through advanced computer calculations. Around 1957, Allan Cormack developed the necessary methods of calculation. In addition to cross-sections of the body, computerized tomography also provides a basis for three-dimensional images.

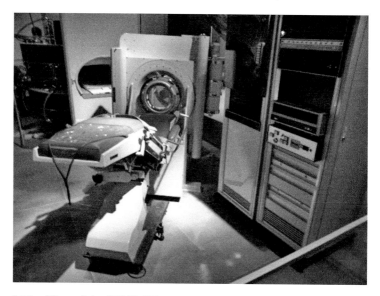

Figure 9.13   The original EMI CT scanner. (commons.en.wikimedia.org)[13]

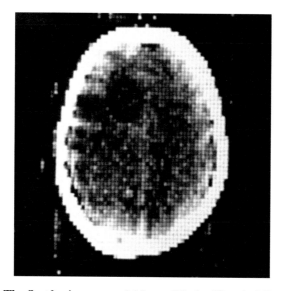

Figure 9.14a   The first brain scan, at Atkinson Morley Hospital, London. First original CT image from the dedicated EMI scanner, October 1971. The patient was a woman with a suspected frontal lobe tumor, visible as a circular dark area on the upper left side. This image has a low-resolution matrix, 80 × 80 pixels. However, in 1971, physicians were fascinated by the ability to see the soft tissue structures of the brain. (Image courtesy: This figure is licensed under the terms of the Creative Commons Attribution 4.0 International License. https://creativecommons.org/licenses/by/4.0/. Credit to the authors: Maier A, Steidl S, Christlein V, et al., editors. Cham [CH]: Springer; 2018.)[14]

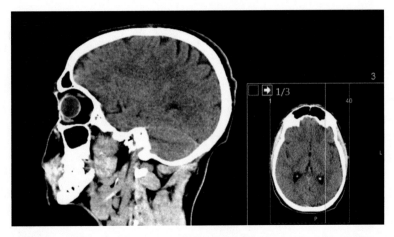

Figure 9.14b   A more contemporary brain scan. (Uploaded by Mikael Häggström, #/media/File: CT of a normal brain, sagittal 28.png, en.wikipedia.org)[15]

Godfrey N. Hounsfield (1919–2004) was a British electrical engineer who developed the first CT scanner. Hounsfield received the Nobel Prize in Medicine in 1979, together with Allan M. Cormac (1924–1998), a mathematician born in South Africa, who developed the algorithm needed to back project the profile collected from the CT scanner and rebuild the image for each slice.

Godfrey Hounsfield built the CT scanner, and Alan Cormac made it possible to reconstruct the radiation profiles the scanner had collected while sampling the radiation profiles from many angles around the body. If X-rays are sent through the body from different angles and registered when they have passed the patient's body, the result will be different attenuation profiles as the X-rays that pass the body will give rise to radiation profiles that are differently attenuated due to the different materials that the X-rays will pass on their way from the patient to the detector. The handling of this complicated scheme of attenuations will be handled of the reconstruction process.

Around 1957, Allan Cormack developed the necessary methods of this calculation. In addition to cross-sections, both gentlemen developed similar technologies almost simultaneously while being in different parts of the world. The first CT was a dedicated head-only scanner. The scanner collected the profiles of the head through a translational movement of the X-ray tube and the sodium iodide (NaI) detector simultaneously along the profile and stored the measurements in the computer memory. Then a new profile of a new angle was scanned/collected and stored. This continued until the X-ray profiles around the patient are all collected.

The first scanner collected 60 different angles around the head before reconstruction took place. The reconstruction took approximately 10 minutes, and you got two 13 mm slices to review on the monitor.

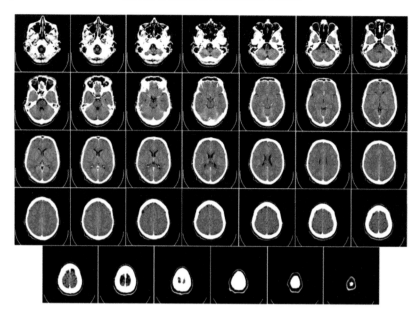

Figure 9.15   Image quality with a modern CT scanner. (Uploaded by Mikael Häggström, en.wikipedia.org)[16]

If I remember right, the matrix size was 80 × 80 pixels in the first model (Figure 9.14a). In the following years, the EMI scanner, as it was called, released several upgrades to improve the image quality, reconstruction speed, and user interface (Figure 9.14b). Moreover, the water-filled box needed for handling the dynamic range of measurements was replaced with wedge filters. Hereby, the patient preparation was largely simplified. In Fig. 9.15 the images from a late CT scanner can be seen.

Personal Anecdote 1

At the time of the introduction of the EMI scanner, I was a young PhD student in Linköping, Sweden, at the Department of Radiation Physics. Together with our research engineer, I was very interested to learn about the potential image quality of this new image modality compared to the conventional X-rays of the time. Our professor helped us and wrote a letter to Godfrey Hounsfield and asked if we could come over to his lab in London and test the image quality with a newly developed tool for this purpose. To all our surprise, we got a very kind letter from Godfrey Hounsfield saying that we were welcome to come and see him and his wonder machine. We could only send one of us to London due to money restrictions, so our research engineer made the trip but with a very detailed protocol for the testing. As we had no experience with the expected image resolution and the contrast resolution, it took us a long week to construct the phantom to be used.

We knew or guessed that the EMI scanner operated at 100 kilovoltages on the X-ray tube and tested if the standard X-ray in our lab could see the difference in contrast between the red and black electrical tape. We could not see any difference in the images. Luckily, we also had access to a mammography X-ray tube, and when we used the low kilovoltage at 25 kV peak, we could see a clear difference between the red and the black tape. With this result, we thought we had a good idea for the manufacturing of something that may well have been the first image-quality phantom for CT.

With this idea, we went to a machine workshop with many packages of red and black electrical tape. Around a pencil, we first wrapped a one-thickness red tape around the pencil and then the same thickness of black tape. For the next turn, we added 2 thicknesses of both red and black tape and so on up to the thickness of 10 turns of tape.

The EMI scanner imaged the brain with consecutive transversal slices, so our phantom was suited to be imaged perpendicular to the tape.

We sent our engineer to London, and the EMI and the homemade phantom functioned perfectly. Godfrey Hounsfield came in person to view the images and inspected the phantom. The results were extremely convincing, and there is no doubt that this also helped to convince our radiologists at the Radiology Department and led to the purchase of an EMI scanner very early in Sweden. We became one of the first hospitals in Sweden to receive an EMI brain CT scanner.

Best of all was that we got two tickets to the Nobel lecture that Hounsfield gave when he received the Nobel Prize. This time, I got a ticket to the lecture. Unfortunately, we did not get a ticket to the Nobel party itself.

Personal Anecdote 2

Working as a hospital physicist those days was exciting, as there were many questions from the radiology staff every day. The neuroradiologist I worked with those days was used to high-resolution images with limited contrast resolution, and now they receive low spatial resolution images with much better contrast resolution.

There were a couple of neuroradiologists that one day came up to me and asked if I could fix the fact that they saw the pixels too clearly and asked if I could get rid of them.

My recommendation as that the people on the staff that used goggles should take them off and give their glasses to their colleagues who do not use glasses.

This very simple image processing advice gave insight but also a lot of laughter for many of the staff.

The introduction of the CT with the EMI scanner for neuro applications had very important clinical implications. The CT brain scans had the effect that the number of neuro-angiographies was substantially reduced. Especially as the image quality was improved rather quickly in a dramatic way from the first-generation CT scanners and the head-only EMI scanner.

The design changed from a rotation/translation mode of data sampling to a rotation-only design, with the detectors arranged together with the X-ray tube in a fan-beam construction, rotating around the patient (see Figures 9.16 and 9.17).

Fan-beam CT: An important development enabling CT to become the prime imaging modality for emergency rooms and a great number of diagnoses and a key modality in advanced surgeries. With this construction, the translational movement could be avoided by letting the X-ray tube and the detector be linked to each other and rotate around the patient (Figure 9.18). The detector unit has a width that sees the whole patient in each view of sampling.

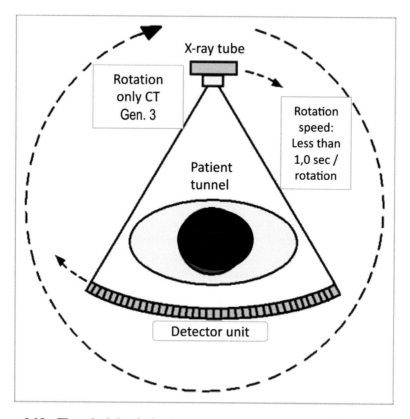

Figure 9.16   The principle of a fan-beam CT scanner. (Modified by Bengt Nielsen.)[17]

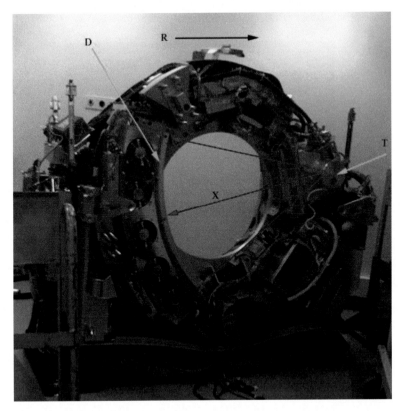

Figure 9.17 This is what is inside a modern CT gantry without a cover. D= detector; T= Tube. (**en.wikipedia.org**)[18]

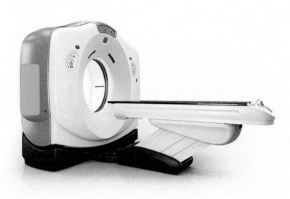

Figure 9.18 This is what the patient will see.

Figure 9.19 shows what the radiologist will see.

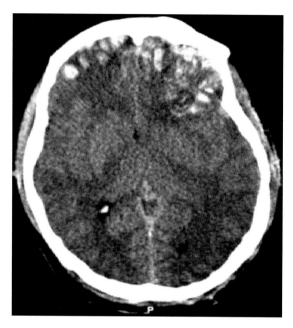

Figure 9.19   Modern CT image, trauma case. (By Rehman T, Ali R, Tawil I, Yonas H [2008]. "Rapid progression of traumatic bifrontal contusions to transtentorial herniation: A case report". Cases journal 1 [1]: 203. doi:10.1186/1757-1626-1-203. PMID 18831756. http://www.casesjournal.com/content/1/1/203 PMC 2566562, CC BY 2.0, https://commons.wikimedia.org/w/index.php?curid=5056582)[19]

The developments from the time of the introduction of the EMI head scanner were very rapid, and newly improved CT scanner models were released every year. It did not take very long until the whole-body version of CTs was out on the market from all vendors.

9.4   Whole-Body Applications with CT

The success of the neuro application of CT made manufacturers quickly start to develop body CTs. The first body CT entered the market in 1976. Yearly upgrades and improvements came from all manufacturers. CT became the main imaging modality in many emergency departments.

Very rapidly, CT became a key imaging tool for radiotherapy planning and led to large improvements in radiotherapy results due to the more precise planning, thereby, saving more healthy tissues during treatment.

Radiotherapy clinics started to invest in their own CT equipment in order to be able to offer an improved service and to be able to do more development work to improve radiotherapy.

The image quality for more modern CT applications can be seen in Figure 9.11 with an example of cardiac imaging and in Figures 9.10 and 9.12 with examples of neuroimaging.

9.5   Different Generations of CT

The first-generation CTs from 1971 had a parallel beam, and the X-ray source was collimated to a pencil beam. The pencil beam was translated to cover the object (in this case, the head), and after the translation was finished, the beam was rotated for the next view/projection to be collected. When all the views and projection profiles were collected, the scan was finished. The whole scan of the brain took approximately five minutes. The data was transferred to a computer where the reconstruction of the image was done. The very first reconstruction method was called back-projection, and it took approximately eight minutes before one slice of the head was ready to be reviewed.

The second-generation CT from 1974 used mini fan beams in order to reduce the number of rotations necessary, and this increased the speed considerably. The scan time was reduced to between 20 seconds and 2 minutes. The second generation was still a head-only scanner.

The third-generation CT from 1975 was a rotate-only CT with a fan-beam X-ray source that covered the whole object in each view, and the X-ray tube rotated simultaneously with the detector. The scan time per slice was one second. This type of scanner won the geometry race, and this geometry is the only construction available today. The third-generation scanners were also all-anatomy units.

The fourth-generation CT from 1976 consisted of a rotating X-ray tube inside a 360-degree stationary detector ring. This construction never became a success, as it was very expensive, plus the fact that it gave a reduction in image quality due to scattered radiation effects. The scan time was one second.

The fifth-generation CT from 1980 was a stationary-stationary scanner. The scanner was dedicated to extremely short scan times, 50 milliseconds. Primarily, cardiac exams were the target. It had no moving parts, but an electron beam electronically moved over a target that generated the X-rays.

The detector was also stationary and had a rather short bit of a ring, as it did not need to cover large volumes, as it mainly focused on scanning the heart. The scan times with the latest conventional CTs (using a normal X-ray tube rotating during the scan) are constantly becoming shorter, and there is hardly a need for the electron beam design. The electron beam scanner has consequently been discontinued.

The limitation of the electron beam CT producing a high flux of X-ray was another limitation that killed this construction. Modern X-ray tubes produce a very high flux of X-ray photons even with the very short scan times of today, and most likely, this will not become a limitation, locking ahead at future CT designs.

9.6   Cone Beam CT

Cone beam computerized tomography systems (CBCT) are a variation of traditional computerized tomography CT systems (Figure 9.20). CBCT systems are used mainly by dental professionals and rotate around the patient, capturing data using a cone-shaped X-ray beam. These data are used to reconstruct a three-dimensional (3D) image of the following regions of the patient's anatomy: dental (teeth); oral and maxillofacial region (mouth, jaw, and neck) (Figure 9.21); and ears, nose, and throat.

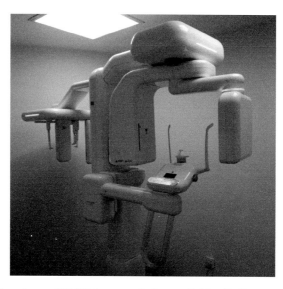

Figure 9.20   Cone beam CT: Highest resolution available. (By Ptrump16 – Own work, CC BY-SA 4.0, https://commons.wikimedia.org/w/index.php?curid=116232460)[20]

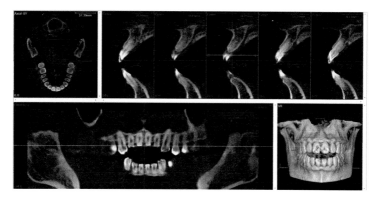

Figure 9.21   Detailed cone beam CT images of the jaw: Panoramic radiograph, axial, sagittal plane of CBCT, 3D reconstruction; highest resolution available. (By Panda 51 – Own work, CC BY-SA 4.0, https://commons.wikimedia.org/w/index. php?curid=37666549)[21]

9.7 Photon-Counting CT: Probably the Sixth-Generation CT

The detector material used in all the earlier models/generations of CTs used several different materials, xenon gas, different scintillating materials, and so on. The common denominator for all previous CT detectors has been that the detector signal in each detector element is integrated during the scan. This has, of course, been functioning well technically but misses a great deal of information from the passage of each photon through the body parts.

With the new-generation CT, using photon counting, it is possible to detect each photon and organize the photons in energy bands. This means that we will be able to measure the attenuation for different energies and, therefore, better differentiate between tissues in different body parts.

Consequently, we will be able to start receiving new information about the different tissues than possible with the multi-energetic photon beam coming from the X-ray tube when passing on its way through the human body. The different energies will be attenuated differently, and this will give us new information.

The information has the potential to be both qualitative and quantitative.

This is possible because of new detector materials being used as well as new and much faster electronics.

Both Siemens and Philips have launched photon-counting products already, and the rest of the manufacturers will move in the same direction one by one.

GE HealthCare has a unit in clinical validation for the moment, in preparation for a product launch probably in 2023 or 2024.

9.7.1 Reality and Expectations for the New Photon-Counting CT

Minimal electric noise: This leads to better image quality for specifically obese patients and in low-dose scans.

Smaller detector pixels: This will greatly improve spatial resolution to improve image quality over conventional CT scanners and help further reduce noise.

No down-weighting of lower-energy photons: This improves image contrast, including iodine contrast–to–noise ratio (CNR).

Intrinsic spectral imaging built into each scan: All photon-counting scans have a spectral CT component because the detector registers photons in different energy bins, allowing them to be accessed in postprocessing to show the image at different energies. These scanners will eliminate the need for dedicated dual-energy CT scanners.

Direct digital detection of photons without a scintillator: Removing the two-step conversion process to convert X-ray photons into visible light helps improve image quality. This also allows photon-counting detectors to differentiate the energy of each photon to enable dual-energy, spectral imaging.

The expectation is that these new CT systems will be able to deliver lower dose, improved spatial resolution, together with better contrast resolution all at the same time. It sounds like a dream without any reality in the real clinical world until now.

Different manufacturers are using different detector materials in their scanners as we know them today.

A photon-counting detector is a detector that registers the interactions of individual photons. By keeping track of the deposited energy in each interaction, the detector pixels of a photon-counting detector record an approximate energy spectrum, making it a spectral- or energy-resolved CT technique.

In contrast, more conventional CT scanners use energy-integrating detectors, where the total energy (generally from many photons as well as electronic noise) deposited in a pixel during a fixed period is registered.

> *Philips Healthcare* is using two different detector materials in order to obtain energy selectivity. The front detector (after the patient) is zinc selenide (ZnSe), and the second detector material is gadolinium oxysulfide (GOS). The low-energy photons are stopped in the front detector, and the photons with higher energy are detected in the rear second detector.
>
> *Siemens Healthineers* is using cadmium telluride in their photon-counting detector. Cadmium telluride and cadmium zinc telluride detectors have the advantage of high attenuation and a relatively high photoelectric-to-Compton ratio for X-ray energies used in CT imaging.
>
> *GE HealthCare*, together with Prismatic Sensors (now GE HealthCare) in Stockholm, is using only one type of photon-counting detector material, namely silicon. Silicon has the advantage of being relatively easy to manufacture, with very high precision, and can also be expanded to deep detectors in order to stop high-energy photons.

With the silicon detector material, the hundreds of millions of photons reaching the detector every second can be counted, and the energies can be registered fast enough in order to make use of not only the number of photons but also the attenuation as a function of the energy of the photons. This will give new and very important spectral information, opening up new, very exciting information that CT never has been able to produce. In the future, this could lead to a whole new range of applications in CT scanning.

Note: This new CT from GE HealthCare is still not commercially introduced, but clinical validation is ongoing.

Which of the three solutions will bring the best clinical imaging and become the preferred solution we will most likely know within a few years?

9.8   Today CT Is the Main Contributor of Radiation Exposure within Diagnostic Imaging

The concept of effective radiation dose has been used to compare the effect that different types of ionizing radiation have on our biology and in relation to the sensitivity of different organs and tissues in our bodies. It turns out that medical imaging is the largest contributor to the population's radiation dose in Sweden. Looking at medical imaging, the technique that gives the highest contribution is CT. This result was obtained from a study in 2005. The same study was repeated in 2018, and the effective radiation dose had doubled. The reason is that many of the standard X-ray examinations have been replaced by CT examinations. The clinical value (i.e., the diagnostic value of a CT examination) was considerably better using CT compared to flat-panel X-rays. Consequently, there is a strong motivation to reduce CT doses as much as possible without degrading the fantastic image quality obtained today, which results in outstanding diagnostic capabilities.

At the same time, there is no way we could live without CT imaging in today's medicine, especially in emergency and trauma medicine.

CT is, for those applications, an indispensable component. Many different techniques have been suggested, tested, and implemented in order to reduce the CT dose without degrading the image quality and maybe even enhancing image quality. Recently, Philips Healthcare introduced IMR (Iterative Model Reconstruction), combined with new computational hardware, which has demonstrated simultaneously significant improvements in image quality and significantly lower dose, with reconstruction times of less than five minutes for a dominating number of the reference protocols.

The evolution to knowledge-based iterative reconstruction algorithms that utilize additional system information to enable significant CT radiation dose reduction and image quality improvement is, at the same time, the next step in CT technology innovation. Although these more advanced algorithms have been used in single-photon emission computerized tomography (SPECT) and positron-emission tomography (PET) for some time, their use in CT was historically limited by long, clinically unacceptable reconstruction times.

Reference List, Chapter 9

1 *Original Slide Made by Bengt Nielsen.* Data from Wikipedia.
2 https://en.wikipedia.org/wiki/Crookes tube
3 https://en.wikipedia.org/wiki/X-ray_tube#/media/File:Xraytubeinhousing_commons.png
4 https://en.wikipedia.org/wiki/X-ray_tube
5 Image Quality in Diagnostic Radiology, Bengt Nielsen, Thesis 1985, Linköping University, Sweden
6 With Courtesy from Medical Collections of Region Skåne. Photographer: Per Bagge.

7 Image Quality in Diagnostic Radiology, Bengt Nielsen, Thesis 1985, Linköping University, Sweden

8 Principle of X-ray tomography, own illustration

9 https://en.wikipedia.org/wiki/X-ray image intensifier

10 https://en.wikipedia.org/wiki/Cerebral_angiography

11 CC BY 2.5, https://commons.wikimedia.org/w/index.php?curid=1694485

12 By Mikael Häggström—own work, CC0, https://commons.wikimedia.org/w/index.php?curid=61405609

13 https://commons.wikimedia.org/w/index.php?search=the+first+EMI+scanner&title=Special:MediaSearch&go=Go&type=image

14 www.ncbi.nlm.nih.gov/books/NBK546157/figure/ch8.fig2/

15 https://commons.wikimedia.org/wiki/File:CT_of_a_normal_brain,_sagittal_28.png#/media/File:CT_of_a_normal_brain, sagittal_28.png. Uploaded by Mikael Häggström

16 https://en.wikipedia.org/wiki/Computed_tomography_of_the_head#/media/File:Computed_tomography_of_human_brain_-_large.png. Uploaded by Mikael Häggström

17 Bengt Nielsen: *Modified Drawing of the Principle of the CT Fan Beam Technique.* Inspired of an image from inside a modern CT gantry. This Figure. 9.17, https://en.wikipedia.org/wiki/Operation_of_computed_tomography#/media/File:Ct-internals.jpg

18 https://en.wikipedia.org/wiki/Operation_of_computed_tomography

19 T Rehman, R Ali, I Tawil, H Yonas, 2008 https://commons.wikimedia.org/wiki/File:Brain_trauma_CT.jpg#/media/File:Brain_trauma_CT.jpg

20 https://en.wikipedia.org/wiki/Cone_beam_computed_tomography

21 https://commons.wikimedia.org/wiki/File:CBCT_image_03.png#/media/File:CBCT_image_03.png

10

MOLECULAR IMAGING

The era of X-ray imaging and CT gave us primarily morphological images of organs and the ability to see details inside organs and biological structures (Figures 10.1 and 10.2).

With physiological images, we could see vascular flows, permeability, and activity in the central nervous system (CNS) and could study different mechanisms in the human body.

Molecular imaging (nuclear medicine [NM] and positron-emission tomography [PET]) is a very important tool in today's medicine, as it will give us functional information about the organ investigated.

Molecular imaging gives us a visual representation, characterization, and quantification of biological processes at the cell and sub-cell levels in living objects. Molecular imaging uses specific molecules as image contrast.

Molecular imaging is said to be a combination of technology and biology and chemistry. Some people say, "Hardware + Wetware + Software."

The starting point of the era of molecular imaging was the introduction of the Anger camera, today called the gamma camera.

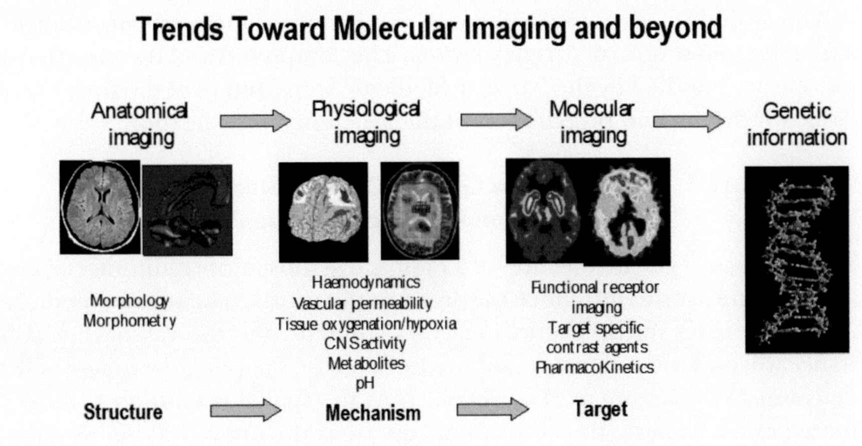

Trends Toward Molecular Imaging and beyond

Anatomical imaging → Physiological imaging → Molecular imaging → Genetic information

Morphology / Morphometry

Haemodynamics / Vascular permeability / Tissue oxygenation/hypoxia / CNS activity / Metabolites / pH

Functional receptor imaging / Target specific contrast agents / PharmacoKinetics

Structure ⇒ Mechanism ⇒ Target

Figure 10.1 The imaging journey toward molecular imaging and beyond. (Image courtesy Bengt Långström. Collaboration between Bengt Långström and Bengt Nielsen.)[1]

DOI: 10.1201/9781003393320-12

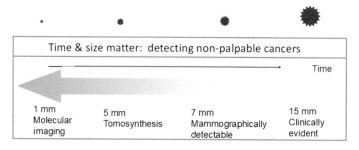

The 1mm challenge: early detection - very important

TRACERS: Do not impact the biology and have no pharmacological effect

Contrast media, used today: Pharmacological effects exists and may impact biology

Figure 10.2   The 1 mm challenge in cancer. (Bengt Nielsen in collaboration with Bengt Långström.)[2]

Hal Oscar Anger (1920–2005) was an American electrical engineer and biophysicist at Donner Laboratory, University of California, Berkeley, known for his invention of the gamma camera.

Before you lie down on the examination table of a gamma camera, you will receive an injection of a compound that will bind to a specific organ or a specific tissue. The compound injected is also labeled with a radioactive isotope in order for the gamma camera to be able to detect the isotope and, indirectly, the organ or tissue where the radioactive substance binds.

The different compounds used during a gamma camera investigation are available from several different vendors. The compound and the radioactive isotope are handled by the Nuclear Medicine Department at the hospital or clinic for dosing and preparation of the functional investigation.

10.1   Principles of a Gamma Camera: Single-Photon Emission Computerized Tomography

The patient will get an injection of a radioactive substance (radiotracer), and after waiting for the substance to spread to the organ to be investigated, the imaging session starts. The gamma rays emitted from the radioactive substance will pass the collimator and hit the detector, sampling the image of the emission from the organ (Figure 10.3). As the spatial resolution is limited for a gamma camera, the emission image from the organ will be overlayed on a CT image in order to be able to locate precisely the emission image in relation to the rest of the body part imaged with the CT.

Today, most gamma cameras are equipped with a CT in order to give improved and accurate localization (Figure 10.4).

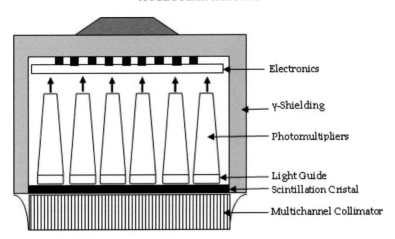

Figure 10.3   Gamma camera. (With courtesy: Imaging and Radioanalytical Techniques in Interdisciplinary Research—Fundamentals and Cuttine Edge Applications, by Faycal Kharfi. © 2013 The Author[s]. Licensee IntechOpen. This chapter is distributed under the terms of the Creative Commons Attribution 3.0 License, which permits unrestricted use, distribution, and reproduction in any medium, provided the original work is properly cited.)[3]

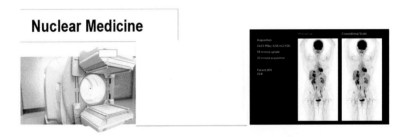

Figure 10.4   Gamma camera and CT for diagnosing organs, such as the kidneys, liver, and lungs. The gamma camera uptake is overlayed on the CT image in order to have a localization that only the CT can offer.

10.2   Positron-Emission Tomography—Functional Studies

PET scanning is based on short-lived isotope emissions following radioactive decay with a positive electron. When the positron meets an electron (with a negative charge), it will be annihilated, and the energy of this annihilation is emitted as two 512 keV gamma rays, with photons almost exactly anti-directional, at 180 degrees (Figure 10.5). These two photons are detected in coincidence by the PET detector (Figure 10.6). This means that only beta-emitting isotopes can be used.

When the radioactive isotope is injected into the body of the patient and the radioactive decay of positrons is emitted, they meet electrons, and

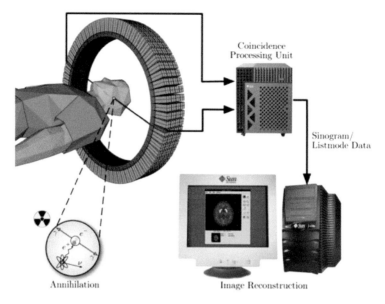

Figure 10.5   The electronics of a PET scanner and ring of a PET during the annihilation processes. (en.wikipedia.org)[4]

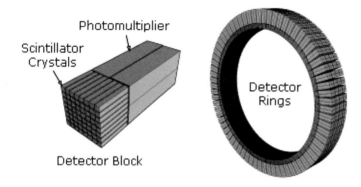

Figure 10.6   The detector scanner is stationary. (en.wikipedia.org)[5]

rather immediately, the annihilation process takes place. The annihilation happens when the emitted positron coming from the used beta-emitting isotope meets its anti-particle, the electron.

Following this event, two anti-directional photons are sent out, and it is these two photons that are detected in two detector elements in a straight line. The duration of the annihilation process is extremely short, and this is why it can be detected in the PET scanner as a coincidence and, hereby, becomes a unique registration belonging to the event in the human body where the radioactive-labeled molecule has resided.

After passing the coincidence circuit, the event is registered, and the point of intersection of the rays from each point of origin of the radiotracer can be established.

After the exam time, all the measurements that have been collected are reconstructed, and an image of the volumes where the radiotracer has been accumulated can be presented. Today, the PET image is always overlayed with a CT image in order to have the exact localization of the different targets of tracer accumulation in relation to the actual body anatomy. The equipment is, therefore, normally called PET/CT (see Figures 10.7, 10.8, and 10.9).

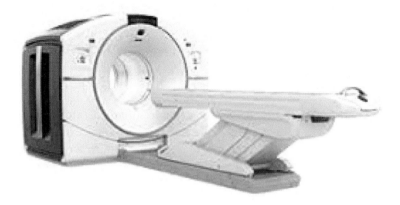

Figure 10.7   Commercial PET/CT scanner.

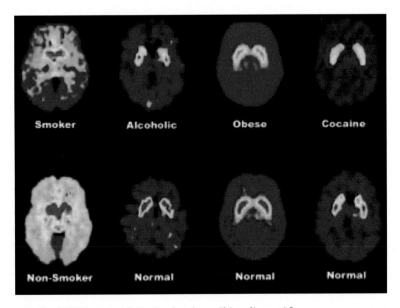

Figure 10.8   PET image of the brain. (en.wikipedia.org)[6]

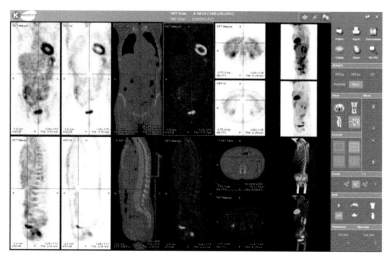

Figure 10.9   PET examples of the body. (en.wikipedia.org)[7]

PET scanning demands the use of suitable molecules that will bind to those organs and locations that are the target for the PET exam.

The molecules are then labeled with a suitable radiotracer before injection into the patient. The labeling exercise is done in a radio chemistry lab for the tracer dose to be adapted to the patient's weight and so on. PET uses radioactive material, and hence, it needs a specially adapted laboratory for this purpose. In addition, the tracer will be injected into humans and, therefore, needs to be handled rigorously, like any injected medicine, with strong regulatory handling. The fact that the tracer is radioactive is, of course, an additional complication.

For labeling PET molecules, many different radioisotopes can be used. In order to have full flexibility with tracer development, you will need to have a cyclotron. Here is where the challenges begin. Tracer centers with full flexibility are expensive and rather staff-demanding units. Hence, today, it is mostly university hospitals that have direct access to a wide range of radiotracers.

You will be able to use PET imaging even if you do not have a cyclotron. In this case, you need to receive delivery of some isotopes from a nearby cyclotron preferably.

Different isotopes have different half-life, and hence, the preferred tracers with a short half-life cannot routinely be transported.

Such an arrangement means that you most likely cannot work with very short half-life tracers like ^{13}C with a half-life of 20 minutes and other endogenous tracers (tracers that are naturally available in our body, and as such, they have minimal side effects). You will, unfortunately, be limited to a smaller number of radiotracers and, hence, also somewhat limited in the type of exams you will be able to offer.

Note: There are more than 1,500 medical cyclotrons in the world used for radio-nuclei production. The PET scanner was developed in 1973. Therefore, the expansion has been rather fast. The driver for the expansion of the technique has, of course, been that PET brings a lot of new value to treatments of severe diseases with high sensitivity but also provides high specificity.

10.2.1 Commonly Used Radiotracers

FDG (fluorodeoxyglucose) has a half-life of ^{18}F = 110 minutes. This is a cyclotron-produced tracer and suits well for distribution to nearby sites due to its relatively long half-life. FDG is probably the most-used isotope today in most parts of the world.

Other important cyclotron-produced radiotracers are on top of ^{11}C with a half-life of 20 minutes, ^{15}O with a half-life of 2 minutes, and ^{13}N with a half-life of 10 minutes. The endogenous radiotracers need to be produced close to the PET scanner due to the very short half-life, as mentioned earlier. The reason that they are interesting is that they are endogenous tracers, meaning that their stable isotope is naturally available in our bodies, and the functionality in the body does not depend if they are radioactive or not.

In addition to the described radiotracers earlier, there are also generator-based radiotracers. One such example is ^{68}Ga, with a half-life of 270 days. If you purchase such a generator, you can use it for more than a year before it must be replaced due to reduced activity.

The challenge is that rather few hospitals around the world are using PET imaging due to the technical demands to invest in and run such a service. In addition, is the manpower and expertise needed for the setup of a full PET service. The present types of cyclotrons have a weight of approximately 40–50 tons, meaning that it has to be placed in the basement of a hospital in most cases.

This, in turn, means that in order to get the tracers to the synthesis and labeling unit, where the molecules will be made radioactive, they will need to be transported as a gas or as a fluid through pipes in the hospital. Alternatively, the radioactive-labeled tracers have to be transported by manpower as ready-to-be-injected doses.

These challenges mean that for PET to become a commodity modality in a medical setting with optimal service, several steps of simplification, automation, and ease of use have to be introduced.

Hence, we are still in the research era of the PET imaging modality, with a lot of development potential, mainly on the radiochemistry side.

An interesting physics historic look is that the positron was theoretically postulated by the English mathematician Paul Dirac during the early 1930s. The Dirac theory is that there must exist a positive electron in order to fulfill the quantum mechanical theory.

Paul Dirac received the Nobel Prize in Physics in 1933, together with Werner Heisenberg and Erwin Schrödinger for their theoretical work in the quantum mechanics theory and the new productive forms of atomic theory.

Personal Anecdote

In 1972, I was a young physicist just about to start my PhD studies. I had the privilege of spending a long summer at CERN, outside Geneva. I worked at the Health Physics Department, and one day, my boss told me that the following day, I should not make any lunch arrangements, as he wanted me to attend an important lunch.

The next day, I met up with him at one of the CERN restaurants at noon, as agreed. When I approached our table with my boss, I immediately recognized Paul Dirac. As a young physicist, this meeting was like meeting the Beatles for a Beatles fan.

For me, Paul Dirac was like a rock star, while his appearance was that of an English gentleman.

It took approximately 50 years before we started to benefit clinically from Paul Dirac and his colleagues Werner Heisenberg and Erwin Schrödinger's theoretical postulates that a positive electron must exist—the positron.

Let's have a look at the different modalities we have available today for early diagnosis.

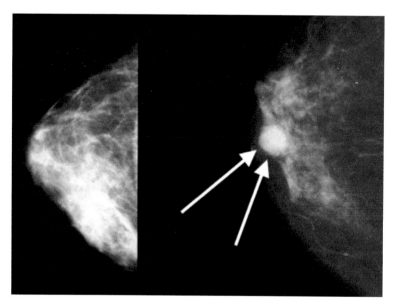

Figure 10.10   Normal mammography image to the left. Mammography image with a breast cancer to the right. Breast cancer detected with mammography. (commons.wikimedia.org)[8]

If we could diagnose cancer very early, already in the molecular phase long before any symptoms arise, there is a better chance that we could avoid serious cancer in the later stage of life. Therefore, more and more diagnostic methods are focusing on the very early signs and prognostic-based methodologies. Molecular medicine tools as well as genetic methods are being developed that eventually will enable the goal of diagnosis before symptoms arise. This will be discussed more in Chapter 18.

Early detection is very important in the case of breast cancer but in fact important for all types of diseases. It gives the chance for therapy to become successful additional odds in the case of cardiovascular disease as well as neurological diseases.

This has led to the development of very sensitive methods, but we must remember that specificity is also an important criterion for future developments.

10.3   Sensitivity and Specificity

Note: MR spectroscopy can only be done on high-field magnets (1.5 T and higher). Not all manufacturers of MRI systems offer this option.

It is fantastic that we can image different healthcare problems with higher and higher sensitivity. The radiologists and the clinicians are educated and learn and practice so that they are able to judge and interpret medical problems from the images. Experience and practice are very critical for the outcome. Most of the modalities we use today are sensitive but rather non-specific. So, for instance, in mammography (Figures 10.11 and 10.12), we

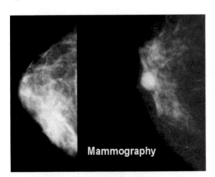

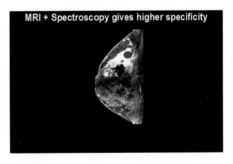

Figure 10.11   Mammography images. The image on the left is normal. The image to the right shows a tumor. From the mammography image you don't know if the tumor is benign or cancer. To find out, a biopsy needs to be taken and the cells analyzed with microscopy. (Original clinical image from en wikipedia.org)[9]

Figure 10.12   This image was obtained with a MRI-unit with spectroscopy, analysing the tissue in the tumor (red area). In case the spectroscopy detects Choline, it is very likely to be a cancer as Choline is a biomarker for cancer. This example shows how the specificity can be increased. (Modified illustration by Bengt Nielsen Original clinical image: en.wikipedia.org)[10]

Note: Not all manufacturers offer a spectroscopy option on their high-field MRIs and the field strength needs to be above 1.5 T.

can see a white, round area that turned out to be cancer. The only way to be sure that this white spot is cancer is to do a biopsy and look at the cells obtained with a microscope.

There are some modalities that can help and increase the specificity: single-photon emission computerized tomography (SPECT) and positron-emission tomography (PET). With radioactive-specific tracers, it is possible to label and inject into the patient and then wait for the molecule with its tracer to reach and bind onto a specific organ or tissue, followed by the imaging session. With this technique, the different imaging techniques could become increasingly more specific. This is the reason why different imaging techniques are combined/integrated. The latest such innovation is the PET/MRI, where the PET shows what we see, and the MRI shows where in the body we are and what nearby organs or tissues we want to avoid in connection with therapeutics after the diagnosis. See more later.

Figure 10.13 shows that the most sensitive imaging modality we have today is PET. The concentrations that PET can measure are in the range of pico to femtomolar (10^{-12}–10^{-15}) concentrations.

We are, consequently, on the way to being able to reach biology with an imaging method.

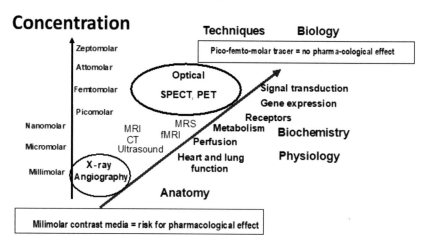

Figure 10.13   Concentrations, Functions, and Technology—sensitivity for different techniques in relation to things we want to detect. (Courtesy by Bengt Långström; collaboration between Bengt Långström and Bengt Nielsen.)[11]

Let's put sensitivity in perspective.

The concentration of the contrast media we use for imaging is in the millimolar range. We know that this can create pharmacological reactions. The fact that the PET radiotracers we use have pico and femtomolar concentrations means these tracers have no pharmacological effect.

10.4   Integration of Two Diagnostic Modalities in the Same Equipment

The key in all diagnostic work is that the methods must provide very sensitive results, but at the same time, preferably, it must also be specific.

In a diagnostic test, sensitivity is a measure of how well a test can identify true positives. The specificity is a measure of how well a test can identify true negatives. For all testing, both diagnostic and screening, there is usually a trade-off between sensitivity and specificity such that higher sensitivities will mean lower specificities and vice versa.[12]

Hence, the integration of different diagnostic equipment into one combined unit is aimed to increase mainly the specificity. Subsequently, I have listed a few of the most common types of diagnostic equipment combinations today.

The integration of a gamma camera with a CT is rather logical, as the spatial resolution of the SPECT is insufficient in case you need precise localization for surgery or need to know if a specific organ is involved or not. As a consequence, modern SPECT cameras (gamma cameras) are all linked with a CT as well.

The modality is called SPECT/CT.

The same goes for positron-emission tomography (PET). The combined modality is called PET/CT. For both the SPECT/CT and the PET/CT, the imaging planes for the two different modalities are shifted and can then be overlayed in exact geometry when the examination is finished. Patient movements between the two registrations can give rise to small distortions.

The latest combined modality is PET/MRI, where the PET camera is fully integrated with the MRI unit so that they have simultaneous registration. The MRI gives the soft tissue and precise geometrical information, while the PET gives specificity through its molecular sensitivity and molecular binding of the tracer injected. PET/MRI has been on the market for approximately 10 years, and there are approximately 150 units worldwide today.

The combination of PET and MRI provides a unique clinical imaging tool with significant applications in biomedical research in small animals. PET/MRI systems for use in humans were first introduced in the year 2010. PET/ MRI has a unique capability to improve both sensitivity and specificity in challenging clinical questions. Since a few years the clinical outcomes have been evaluated for several new applications using the two modalities simultaneous.

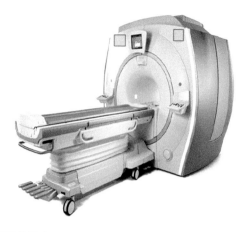

Figure 10.14   PET/MR1—example 1.

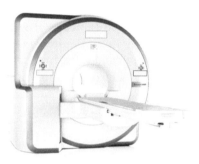

Figure 10.15   PET/MR1—example 2.

The advantages of a combined PET/MR (Figures 10.14 and 10.15), as compared to conventional imaging methods, include the following:

- Lower radiation dose from PET/MRI compared to PET/CT.
- Simultaneous multi-modality preclinical imaging.
- Excellent soft tissue contrast.
- Plenty of tracers available for PET.
- Good visualization, quantification, and translational studies.
- Cryogen-free magnets will highly reduce infrastructure needs in the future.
- Improved disease specificity is expected with the combination of MRI and PET.

The use of PET/MRI in neurology and neuro-oncology is mainly because of its ability to provide complementary functional, morphological, molecular, and pathological-physiological information related to the brain. The PET part of the combination of the two modalities will also be able to bring more specificity to the diagnosis.

10.5   Applications of Combined/Simultaneous PET/MRI

Combined PET/MRI has found applications mainly in oncology. It allows high-resolution imaging of the four key steps in cancer formation; namely, apoptosis (programmed cell death) resistance, cancer angiogenesis, tumor proliferation, and cancer metastasis.

PET/MRI finds use in several key clinical as well as research applications in the fields of neurology, cardiology, and cancer. Combined/fully integrated PET/MRI imaging modality enables simultaneous multifunctional and anatomical imaging in small animals, which greatly impacts biomedical imaging in research and clinical settings.

10.6   Ultrasound: An Imaging Modality Used for Real-Time Examinations

Ultrasound is sound waves with frequencies higher than the upper audible limit of human hearing. Ultrasound is not different from normal, audible sound in its physical properties, except that humans cannot hear it. This limit varies from person to person and is approximately 20 kilohertz (20,000 hertz) in healthy young adults. Ultrasound devices operate with frequencies from 20 kHz up to several gigahertz.

Ultrasound is used in many different fields. Ultrasonic devices are used to detect objects and measure distances. Ultrasound imaging or sonography is often used in medicine. In the non-destructive testing of products and structures, ultrasound is used to detect invisible flaws.

Since the invention of ultrasound imaging, ultrasound as a modality has improved extremely fast and developed to be one of the high-tech equipment used in our hospitals. The fact that you can easily take the ultrasound unit to the patient is a very big advantage.

Personal Anecdote

During the late 1970s, when I was working as a hospital physicist, we were delivered a brand-new ultrasound unit to be used for general abdominal imaging. At the inauguration and demonstration of the ultrasound unit, I was standing next to our chief abdominal radiologist. This was when body imaging with CT was the prime modality. The radiologist called upon me and whispered, "Bengt, can you see anything?" I had to answer him that truthfully, I could not see anything either. Probably we were not trained enough those days on ultrasound. Today, the developments are both on the image quality and also on its very different transceiver technique and the wider range of frequencies used. Ultrasound is probably the imaging modality that has made the most rapid developments and growth. Today's handheld ultrasound units are also moving ultrasound into primary care use. When it comes to visibility, also for a layman, we know that it is hard not to discover if it is a boy or a girl rather early during pregnancy.

The ultrasound units depicted in Figures 10.16, 10.17, and 10.18 are all units for different purposes. Figure 10.16 is a standard/common ultrasound

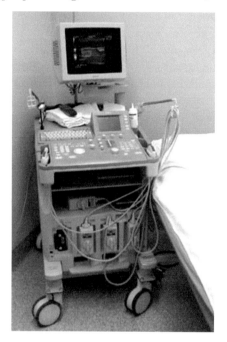

Figure 10.16   Example 1: Standard/common type of ultrasound unit for general purpose.

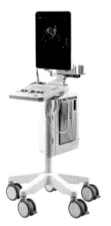

Figure 10.17   Example 2: Neurosurgical ultrasound.

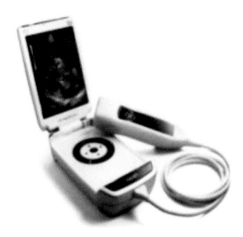

Figure 10.18   Example 3: Handheld ultrasound.

unit for general purposes. The unit in Figure 10.17 is a specialized ultra-sound unit for real-time ultrasound during neurosurgery. Finally, the unit in Figure 10.18 is a handheld ultrasound unit for general purposes but is very efficient for cardiovascular purposes. As it can be carried in your pocket and be battery-driven, it is used for acute purposes and has also been introduced in primary care.

A big advantage of ultrasound is that it does not use ionizing radiation, like several other modalities.

10.7   The Newest in Ultrasound

Engineers at MIT have created an ultrasound patch that can provide long-term ultrasound imaging of internal organs and structures. The device contains a rigid piezoelectric probe array and uses an underlying layer of elastomer-covered hydrogel in lieu of the gel applied to the skin during conventional ultrasound procedures. At just the size of a postage stamp, the ultrasound patch is highly portable and less expensive than conventional ultrasound technologies. The current iteration of the device requires a wired connection to view the images, but the researchers are working to make the device wireless and report that in the future the technology may be suitable for patients to take home and apply themselves.

At present, ultrasound imaging requires a clinician or technician to apply a messy gel and hold a probe against the skin to obtain images of the under-lying organs. This is clearly impractical for long-term imaging, and it also requires expensive equipment and the need to attend a clinic or hospital. To address this, these researchers have created a small wearable patch that can look inside the body for up to 48 hours.

Previously, researchers have attempted to develop wearable ultrasound technology, with mixed success. "Wearable ultrasound imaging tool would have huge potential in the future of clinical diagnosis," said Chonghe Wang, another researcher involved in the study. "However, the spatial resolution and imaging duration of existing ultrasound patches is relatively low, and they cannot image deep organs."

To achieve better ultrasound resolution, the researchers paired rigid transistors with a sticky layer that can easily attach to the user's skin. This prevents the transistors from shifting position with respect to each other but maintains appropriate skin contact. The hydrogel layer at the bottom of the patch allows sound waves to propagate through, and it is enclosed with an elastomer layer that prevents the gel from drying out.

This new technology is looking very interesting and would have many clinical applications.

10.8   Summary of the 20th Century

Looking back to the 20th century, a few things are worth remembering:

- Many new vaccines were developed during the 20th century. What led to these advances?
- Most vaccines in use today were developed by techniques that were pioneered more than 100 years ago and do not represent the full potential of the field.
- Methods for growing viruses in the laboratory led to rapid discoveries and innovations, including the creation of vaccines for polio.
- Researchers targeted many other common childhood diseases, such as measles, mumps, and rubella, and vaccines for these diseases reduced the disease burden with great success.
- Innovative techniques now drive vaccine research, with recombinant DNA technology and new delivery techniques leading scientists in new directions. Disease targets have expanded, and some vaccine research is beginning to focus on non-infectious conditions, such as addiction and allergies.

Several new surgery techniques and transplants were introduced:

- The use of X-rays as an important medical diagnostic tool spread over the globe very quickly, and this meant that a very good base for diagnosing diseases was established through imaging.
- In the past century, several technologies have had a significant impact on surgical practice. These include electrosurgery in the early 20th century; practical endoscopy beginning in the 1960s; and laser surgery, computer-assisted surgery, and robotic surgery developed in the 1980s.

Many new important imaging technological discoveries entered the market and significantly enhanced and changed diagnostic capabilities dramatically:

- An important new modality within radiology was CT, wherein for the first time, an imaging modality was connected to a computer, where the final image was a back-projected/reconstructed image. The sampled data from the CT's ray profile measurement of the patient in combination with an algorithm gave, in fact, quantitative information and not only a qualitative image that needed to be interpreted by a radiologist.

- In the very beginning, using the EMI head scanner, the pixels in the 80×80 matrix were rather disturbing for the radiologist. This is never any problem with today's scanners with a very high spatial resolution (very small pixel size and matrix size of 512×512 up to 1024×1024). Maybe more important for the radiologists is that the contrast resolution increased as well, leading to far better discrimination between different tissues in the body. Today, the signal-to-noise ratio is very high as well.

- The other breakthrough in this century was the introduction of the MRI. The MRI modality is still under strong continuous development, despite being available for almost 50 years.

Personal Anecdote

During my time as a hospital physicist, the staff that worked on our EMI scanner came to me and asked if I could, in some way, take away the visibility of the pixels. The first EMI scanner had a matrix of 80×80 pixels. My recommendation became a very big joke in the department. I recommended that the radiologists with glasses take them off or move backward from the screen when they read the EMI images and those without glasses borrow a pair of glasses from a colleague or move away from the screen. A very effective and certainly cheap form of image processing.

The choice of imaging modality for diagnosing a specific disease is dependent on the disease and the diagnostic question (Figure 10.19). The availability of the preferred diagnostic tools is also an important parameter. All hospitals and clinics cannot have every possible technique at hand 24/7, including the specialist that needs to interpret the images and propose the treatment, every day of the year. The same is also valid when it comes to therapeutic equipment and/or the right type of surgeon. These questions belong to the healthcare system and how healthcare is organized.

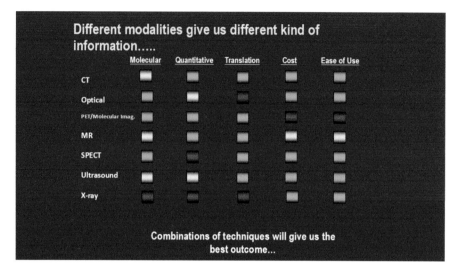

Figure 10.19   The different imaging modalities we use give us different information. Light-gray square means the modality is good for the task. A dark-gray square means the modality is not the best for the task. A black square means that the modality is not suited for the task. (From Bengt Nielsen.)[13]

Note: When I worked as a hospital physicist, there was always a discussion from the administration about the cost and the motivation for investing in a new technology or modality. The administration always wanted or hoped that a new modality would and could replace an older one. The fact of the matter is that no modality has been replaced so far. All the modalities are moving forward with new features and improved image quality. Consequently, even when major development is being made, the conclusion is the same: We need them all in order to serve our citizens with early diagnosis. Each modality gives different and unique information that gives, and will be able to give, specific information needed for diagnosis in order to make the treatment effective.

At the same time, the healthcare officials and the hospital management need to administer the costs, which admittedly must be a challenge.

10.8.1   Thoughts on the 19th- and 20th-Century Developments in Medicine and Medical Technology

The developments in medicine and medical technology during the 20th century have been enormous. The world has also seen huge developments during the 19th century, but what was seen in technological advances in the 20th century is clearly amazing.

My analysis showed that, of 125 projects that came into clinical usage, 53 were technology driven. For the 19th century, the figure was 21 developments, of which 2 were technology projects: the stethoscope and the X-ray. In percentage, 42%, in relation to 9%. These accelerated technological developments within medicine happening from the 20th century will most likely continue at the same speed, and it is more likely to accelerate further in the future.

The outlook on the intense pace of medical technology development and the strong link to medical progress is here to stay and will most likely be accelerated.

10.9 Magnetic Resonance Imaging

The era of magnetic resonance imaging (MRI) started rather early with the introduction of nuclear magnetic resonance (NMR) spectroscopy. Nuclear magnetic resonance was developed in 1945 by two American scientists, Felix Bloch (1905–1983) and Edward M. Purcell (1912–1997), who were awarded the 1952 Nobel Prize in Physics for their work.

The Swiss scientist Richard Robert Ernst was awarded the 1991 Nobel Prize in Chemistry for contributions to the development of the method of high-resolution nuclear magnetic resonance (NMR) spectroscopy. Richard Ernst was the scientist that developed the technique to a level that made it an important step forward in chemistry.

The principle behind NMR is that many nuclei have a spin, and all nuclei are electrically charged. If an external magnetic field is applied, an energy transfer is possible between the base energy and a higher energy level (generally, a single energy gap).

The principle of NMR spectroscopy involves three sequential steps:

1. The alignment (polarization) of the magnetic nuclear spins in an applied, constant magnetic field, B_0 (B-zero).
2. The perturbation (alteration) of this alignment of the nuclear spins by a weak oscillating magnetic field, usually referred to as a radio-frequency (RF) pulse.
3. The detection and analysis of the electromagnetic waves emitted by the nuclei of the sample as a result of this perturbation.

Biochemists use NMR to identify proteins and other complex molecules. Besides identification, NMR spectroscopy provides detailed information about the structure, dynamics, reaction state, and chemical environment of molecules. The most common types of NMR are proton and carbon-13 (^{13}C) NMR spectroscopy, but it is applicable to any kind of sample that contains nuclei with a spin.

NMR spectra are unique for a specific nucleus and well-resolved, analytically tractable, and often highly predictable for small molecules. Different functional groups are obviously distinguishable, and identical functional groups with differing neighboring substituents still give distinguishable signals. NMR has largely replaced traditional wet chemistry tests, such as color reagents or typical chromatography, for identification.

A disadvantage is that a relatively large amount, 2–50 mg, of a purified substance is required. There are ways to overcome this drawback, but they fall outside the aim of this book.

Let's focus on MRI.

The imaging modality of magnetic resonance started with the development by Raymond Damadian in 1980 when the first MRI full-body scanner was built. It was nicknamed the Indomitable (unbeatable). This development started a fantastic and still ongoing development of the new imaging modality, MRI.

10.9.1   The Short, Easy, and Popular Version
of the MRI Principles

The patient is placed in an MRI unit, which has a strong magnet with a static magnetic field that covers/surrounds the entire body part that should be examined. The strength of the magnetic field of an MRI scanner is very much stronger than the earth's magnetic field that is in the range from: (25–65 microtesla, μ T).

The field strength of the commercial magnets goes from 0.5 T all the way up to 7 T. Some research groups are already talking about potential wholebody MRI units of 11 Tesla.

The human body consists predominately of water, approximately 78%. A water molecule is built by two hydrogen (H) atoms and one oxygen (O) atom, H_2O. MRI imaging is focusing on the hydrogen nucleus. This is the proton, and the proton is a magnetic elementary particle.

Note. When we looked at X-ray imaging, the focus was on the interaction of the radiation with the electrons surrounding the nucleus of the atoms.

In a MRI unit the magnetism is due to nuclear magnetic resonance, and in the body, all the small nuclei are pointing in all directions when no external magnetic field is applied to the body. When the patient goes into the MRI unit, all the proton's spins in the body will align with the static magnetic field. The sampling of data starts with a radio wave and is introduced (a perturbation) into the body part to be imaged, and the energy introduced is absorbed by the protons. The proton spins will be tilted at a certain degree, depending on the amount of energy given by the radio wave.

When the radio wave is switched off, the protons will start returning to their original position while sending out weak radio waves that will be registered by the MRI electronics to be used by the reconstruction electronics of the MRI unit.

For registration of the position/orientation of the different proton spins, three different gradient coils are used along the X, Y, and Z axes. These gradient coils add to the static magnetic coil and are turned on and off continuously during an MRI exam.

These on-and-off switches of the gradients create the characteristic and repeating noise you can hear when you are in an MRI scanner. After the sampling of all the data, the MRI image is reconstructed and finally presented to the radiologist for interpretation.

During the 1980s, the first MRI exams were done in the United States and in the United Kingdom.

In 2003, the chemist Paul Lauterbur and the physicist Peter Mansfield received the Nobel Prize in Physiology or Medicine for their work on the MRI.

The fact that Raymond Damadian did not get the Nobel Prize for the MRI made him very upset, and a large campaign against the Nobel Committee was started. As recently as 2021, the thing came up, and the Nobel Committee still defended the decision they made many years back.

Dr. Raymond Damadian died in the fall of 2022.

The basic principles of magnetic resonance imaging are not so easy for a layman to understand.

A more scientific description of the magnetic resonance imaging techniques and MRI's potential can be found in the primer *Basic Principles of MRI* from 1988, written by Dr. Paul Keller, with a foreword by Felix Wehrli.

This primer can be difficult to obtain, but there are plenty of newer books available on MRI physics and the basic principles of MRI by many publishers. These books will also cover many of the newer applications and techniques developed and clinically introduced.

The continuous developments and growing number of clinical applications for the MRI modality, including new organ-specific techniques and continued improvement in speed and image quality, have been amazing and continue to excite us year after year. The fact that the MRI does not use ionizing radiation is an important argument for its usage and continued development.

10.10   Instrumentation

The magnets in the early days of the MRI were mostly of permanent magnet type. They were very expensive, and their magnetic field strength was rather low. The other challenge in the early days was that the permanent magnet weight was very high, and this was a challenge when you want to put an MRI in a hospital building unless you could place it in the basement. The image quality of the MRI is very much depending on the homogeneity of the magnet within the imaging volume and the field strength of the magnet. Consequently, the magnet choice moved very quickly into strong superconducting magnets.

Why has the MRI become such an important medical imaging modality?

The two clinical examples in Figures 10.20 and 10.21 are used to give the readers a glimpse of the typical clinical insight and the image quality that MRI imaging can give our clinicians under standard clinical conditions.

The MRI is undergoing steady development, and we have not seen it slow down the last 10 years and we do not expect it to slow down within foreseeable times. New improved techniques are introduced year after year enabling improved image quality and at the same time with reduced scan times and reduced reconstruction times. Both these images (10.20 and 10.21) are obtained with superconditivity magnets with fieldstrength 1,5T.

The fact that the MRI modality does not use any ionizing radiation is an important factor for the potential developments and future new applications.

10.10.1 Permanent Magnets

Raymond Damadian started the company Fonar, and they built whole-body MRI scanners based on very heavy permanent magnets.

In Sweden, the first of these magnets was installed at the University Hospital in Lund in 1984. It demanded huge floor reinforcements due to the weight of the magnet. My memory tells me that the weight was around 80 tons (maybe my memory slips here, my apologies). Nevertheless, the permanent magnet technology in the early days of the MRI was very heavy, and substantial reinforcement of the floor was needed at most hospitals.

10.10.2 Superconductivity

Superconductivity is the property of certain materials to conduct direct current (DC) electricity without energy loss when they are cooled below a critical temperature (referred to as T_c). These materials also expel magnetic fields as they transition to the superconducting state. The traditional way of getting into the superconductivity domain has been to cool down the wires in the imaging magnets with the use of liquid helium. By using niobium/titanium or niobium/tin surrounded by copper, you can reach 10 Kelvin (–263°C). The drawback of using liquid helium is the cost and the fact that helium is an inert gas and has also become rare and hence the price of liquid helium has increased.

10.10.3 Superconducting Magnets Operating at a Higher Temperature Than –273°C

New materials that can reach superconductivity at higher temperatures are becoming available, which will reduce the cost and the hazard and

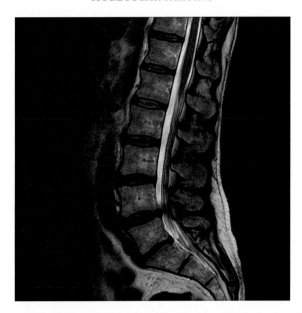

Figure 10.20   MRI of a lumbar spine with degeneration, pre-hemilaminectomy L4–5 (sagittal FRFSE). (https://commons.wikimedia.org/wiki/File:SAGITTALFRFSE-)[14]

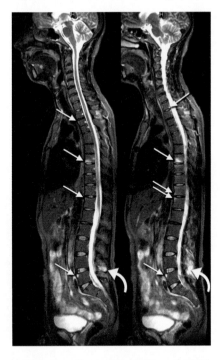

Figure 10.21   A 30-year-old male patient with confirmed AS (duration of pain 7 years), lumbar spine (arrows). There are inflammatory lesions in the spinous process. Sagittal STIR images show inflammatory lesions in the thoracic spine. Annotated MRI shows L4 (curved arrow).[15] (commons.wikimedia.org/w/index.php?curid=52791042, Ptrump16, CC BY-SA-4.0 https://creativecommons.org/licenses/by-)

improve the safety of using liquid helium. This will change the very difficult installations of superconducting magnets and the safety regulations around the liquid helium refilling and quench risks.

The MRI system in Figure 10.22a, b is a superconducting magnet (Figure 10.23) but it uses a material for the generating coils to become superconductive at a higher temperature than 273 Kelvin, resulting in no need for cooling with liquid helium. This makes the installation and running cost much lower and the magnet very much easier to site in an hospital setting.

As you can see from the clinical image, the image quality is excellent even if the field strength is only 0.5 T. The acquisition time is longer than for a 1.5 T or higher field strength in order to get comparable image quality.

This technique and others will, in a positive way, make MRI available in clinics and smaller hospitals, which is a very welcome development for our healthcare systems around the world.

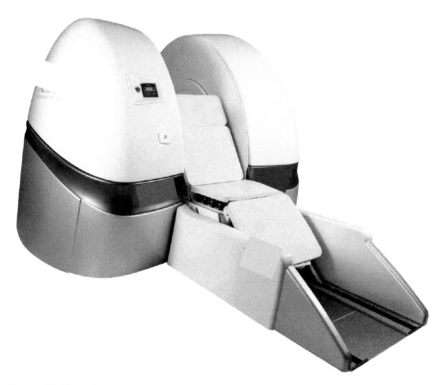

Figure 10.22a   An open system with a superconducting magnet. Diagnostics can be done in standing, sitting, or lying-down position. (Image courtesy: Silvia Fregato, ASG Superconductors SpA.)[16]

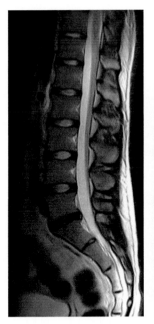
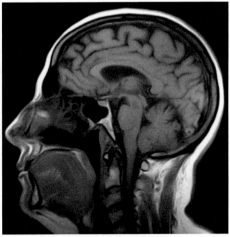

Figure 10.22b Spine image: 5 mm, SE 4.27 min. Head image: 4 mm, FIR PD 4.27 min. (Image courtesy: Silvia Fregato, ASG Superconductors SpA.)[17]

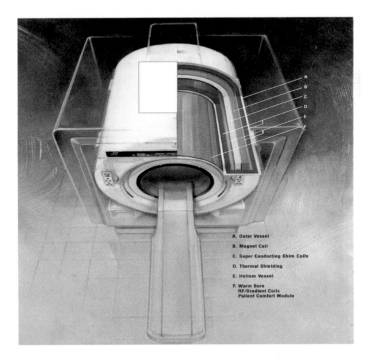

Figure 10.23 Superconducting magnet and its construction.

10.10.4   Latest Magnet Techniques

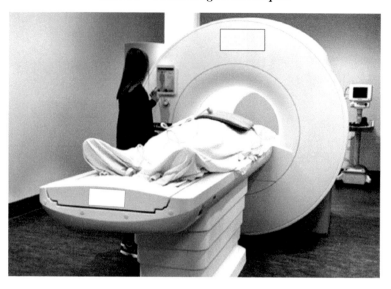

Figure 10.24   Magnetic field strength: 0.55 Tesla. The closed magnet compartment contains only 7 liters of helium. There is no need for a refill within the lifetime of the unit. There is no need for a quench tube in the examination room. Note the extra-large patient bore.

10.10.5   New Electromagnetic Magnet Designs Enabling New and Interesting Applications

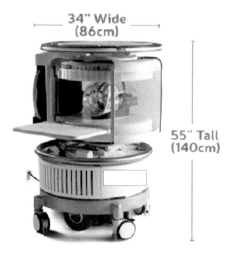

Figure 10.25   Mobile/transportable MRI is now a reality. The magnet can come to the patient.

The magnet designs earlier show how magnetic resonance imaging technology continues to change and has developed since the start, in the 1980s. The magnetic field strength has continued to increase from 0.5 Tesla (T) all the way to 7 Tesla (Figure 10.24). The most common field strengths have become 1.5 T, and lately, the 3.0 T magnets have become a commodity.

The 7 Tesla magnets are still mainly used for research purposes. There are approximately 75,000 MRIs around the world. The majority of these are superconductive 1.5 T magnets.

There are new trends coming into play right now. Most likely, the reduced installation and running costs will drive new technologies and practices in MRI and the general pattern of imaging within a Radiology Department. Increased use of MRI can be expected.

The continued striving for higher and higher field strengths is probably going to fade out or at least flatten somewhat. The present trends are moving in two different directions.

One direction is toward superconducting magnets, with virtually no need for cooling with liquid helium or at least very low helium consumption. This fact has two important implications.

Firstly, it would mean that siting preparation of MRIs in hospitals would be dramatically simplified, and hence, the siting costs will be significantly reduced. All the large companies are now moving in this direction, which means that MRI will become cheaper to install and operate.

Secondly, today, the demand for superconductivity without the need for He cooling (using higher-temperature superconductivity) is opening new avenues.

Instead, the magnet container of the unit can be a closed system and need only less than 7 liters of liquid helium.

Due to the fact that there is no need for refills, as is the case for all older superconductive MRI units, means reduced downtime and that they can also be installed in much smaller rooms.

Moreover, there will be no need for a quench pipe from the magnet toward the outside of the hospital. A considerable simplification and, thereby, a huge cost saving. The guess is that MRIs will become more and more dominant soon and spread into smaller hospitals and smaller clinics (Figure 10.25).

10.10.6 Application-Specific MRI Developments

As the MRI modality becomes more and more developed, specialized or dedicated MRIs have been developed (Figure 10.26). Despite the fact that the more generalized systems can image everything in the human body, it can be an economic advantage for a clinic specialized in a few main applications to look for a dedicated system.

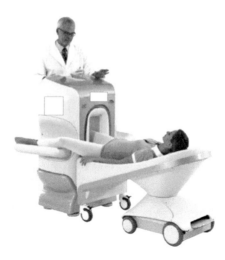

Figure 10.26   Specialized/dedicated MRI for foot, leg, and knee.

It can be expected that the market segment, with a specialized system, will increase along with MRI techniques becoming a commodity within healthcare.

10.10.7   Diagnostic Equipment for Humans Can Also Be Used for Diagnosis in Animals

In the horse-riding community, both speed racing and jumping competitions are huge sports and a big business with betting and so on. The horses in these competitions are very expensive and need medical attention, very much like we people need doctors now and then. When I was at GE HealthCare and responsible for the MRI business, we often got odd requests. We had a permanent rather open magnet dedicated to claustrophobic patients. One day, we received a request from a veterinary hospital in Sweden. They wanted an MR unit where they could image all types of animals from small birds or rabbits all the way up to a full-sized horse. None of the smaller animals, like cats and dogs, were any problem, but a horse is a bit of a challenge to get into an MR machine.

The following is how the challenge ended.

Personal Anecdote

When GE HealthCare sold the first animal MRI scanner to an animal hospital in Sweden, the veterinary team wanted to see a couple of investigations, and the team went for a visit to a veterinary clinic in Spain. There, they saw an examination of a racehorse that had a muscular injury. They were very impressed with the exam when the team managed to get the horse under anesthesia into the MR scanner. However, they were very disappointed with the handling method of the horse. It was dragged sleeping/under anesthesia on a tarpaulin. The whole clinic team had to be called to help move the horse onto the tarpaulin, as the weight of the horse was substantial.

The Swedish veterinary team wanted to buy the MR under the condition that a type of transport table was constructed in order to get the horse to sleep on it and then be able to dock the table to the MR scanner. The demand was that one nurse should be able to maneuver the table with the horse and position the magnet.

It was not so easy to build the table due to the weight of a horse and at the same time make it so flexible that a couple of nurses could maneuver the table with a sleeping horse and dock it to the magnet. The constructor of the table was inspired when he saw a loading of flight containers when he was waiting in an airplane going out of Stockholm. He saw how easily a staff moved a large and presumable heavy container into an aircraft. This is how the design of the table to move and position a horse into an MR unit became a reality.

10.11   What Is a Quench?

Superconductive, high-field MRI systems are basically giant electromagnets. The majority of them operate at 1.5 Tesla, which is equal to 15,000 Gauss, or approximately 30,000 times the earth's magnetic field. This is enough magnetic power to lift a car or to produce miraculous diagnostic images without ionizing radiation. The material that makes these magnets so powerful is liquid helium, which will take the resistance in the windings around the magnet down to zero. This effect is called superconductivity, which means that the electrical current flows continuously if (and this is essential) the liquid helium is maintained at a steady $-273.15°C$.

When a quench happens, a part of the magnet loses the cooling, and the magnet starts to heat up. Thereafter, due to the temperature rise, liquid helium starts moving from the liquid phase to helium gas. This is the reason that all MRIs so far have a helium gas exhaust pipe (often, it is called a quench tube) for the helium gas to be led outside the diagnostic room and further outside the hospital into free air. Helium gas will push out the oxygen in the air we breathe, and consequently, this will be life-threatening.

Personal Anecdote

When I was responsible for the Swedish branch of GE HealthCare, we had four magnets at Karolinska Hospital. I was in my car and was listening to the radio. Suddenly, there was an urgent news interruption about a gas accident near the main entrance of Karolinska Hospital. I did not react, but it only took seconds before I got a call on my mobile telling me that the MRI unit at the radiology department just above the main entrance had quenched. Now, I made the connection and agree that it is rather dramatic (plus, it is also very expensive) when 1,700 liters of liquid helium expands 13 times and comes out of the quench pipe into the open air. The personnel were rather calm but asked me when they could get a refill of 1,700 liters of liquid helium. Their booking list for exams was very long. If I remember correctly, we made this happen within a few days after the quench.

10.12   Installation Requirements for MRI

There are many considerations when installing an MRI unit in a hospital, especially today when most magnets are 1.5 Tesla or higher. In the exam room, special precautions need to be taken by the personnel and the patient. No magnetic materials are allowed inside the exam room. During the years since the introduction of MRI, many accidents have happened, unfortunately. Image quality will be impacted in case any even very small elements will be brought into the bore or close to the bore. In 2019, a person to be imaged was in the bore of a mobile magnet van unit in the north of Sweden. The nurse that handled the patient approached the patient's bed while wearing a metal vest normally used for training purposes and was dragged toward the magnet with huge strength. The patient was not hurt, but the nurse ended up in the intensive care unit.

Most accidents have happened when cleaners or service staff brought magnetic tools into the exam room without knowing or considering the risks. Some accidents have had deadly outcomes.

With very accurate information and routines, together with metal detectors to screen patients, these accidents can be avoided or at least heavily reduced.

When installing an MRI unit, there are other needs and considerations to think about. The magnetic field must be contained inside the exam room, and therefore, there needs to be magnetic shielding in the walls, including on the floor and the ceiling.

Without this magnetic shielding, it would be dangerous or risky to be in the exam room.

The signals collected in the MRI during a scan are very weak. Therefore, the MRI unit needs to be shielded from outside radiofrequency signals as well.

We all realize that installation costs for MRI can become considerable with present technical standards. The new way of cooling for superconductivity will eventually make the installation costs reasonable. This could make the MRI modality a leading modality in healthcare, looking ahead. The number of MRIs will then start to grow from the present level of approximate units worldwide today.

10.13   Different MRI Designs: Pros and Cons

The early permanent magnets were very heavy, and it meant that they were difficult to site into many Radiology Departments, as the floors needed strengthening.

The weight concerns, together with the drive for the very best image quality, moved the MRI segment toward superconducting magnets with lower weight and considerably improved image quality. The weight was lower, but other issues increased with the move toward superconducting magnets. Superconductivity means the need for cooling down the magnet to approximately $-273.15°C = 1$ Kelvin (K).

At this level, there is virtually no molecular motion and no transfer of energy among molecules, at which a thermodynamic system has the lowest energy possible. To cool down a magnet to zero degrees Kelvin, you need many liters of cooling media. There are not too many choices for cooling a magnet but to use liquid helium. Between 1,500 and 2,000 liters of liquid helium is needed to cool an MRI magnet.

New magnet technology on the way out on the market:

- Only 7 liters of liquid helium
- Sealed-for-life magnet design
- No quench pipe
- Significantly reduced life cycle cost

Some vendors use a new, highly efficient micro-cooling technology that requires just 7 liters of liquid helium for cooling, instead of the 1,500 liters that conventional magnets use.

This tiny amount of liquid helium is placed in the magnet and fully sealed during manufacturing, enclosing the precious gas for the rest of its life. No liquid helium can escape. This reduces potential long interruptions to MR services due to helium issues and eliminates helium refill costs during the magnet's lifetime.

Globally, it is estimated that there were about 55 000 MRI machines in the world, as of the year 2007. With a growth of 2,500 new units being produced yearly and sold/installed, we would estimate the number of units today of approximately 90 000 MRI units worldwide.

The expectations are that the volume will continue to grow. The helium-free concept will most likely increase this growth further, as there are many places around the world where it is impossible to get large volumes of helium delivery at present. The use of new materials in the coils generating the magnetic field by obtaining superconductivity at higher temperatures will add to the growth and expansion of magnetic resonance imaging.

The maximum field strength so far reported with the new cooling technique is 1.5 T. If there are challenges using the new cooling technique with the higher field strengths, like 3 Tesla and higher, it is uncertain at this point, or maybe, it is a manufacturing secret.

10.14   Diagnostic Equipment Dedicated to the Brain: Electroencephalography

Electroencephalography (EEG) is a way to study/measure our brain activity. By connecting electrodes to the scalp, the electrical activity can be measured.

It is, therefore, a noninvasive examination. EEG is used, for instance, when epilepsy is in question or when in connection with cramp situations.

EEG is also used today in combination with functional imaging with MRI, fMRI. The fMRI measures the small changes in blood flow when we are using our brains. fMRI is, therefore, since there is a coupling between brain activity and increased blood flow, an indirect method of brain neuronal activity.

The patient can be asked to do a certain brain activity under the magnet while the EEG is being sampled in parallel with MR images being obtained dynamically. This is an exciting capability for brain researchers, as it combines two worlds: The EEG will measure the electrical activity of the brain in a certain area with high temporal resolution, and it is the direct measurement of neuronal activity.

The fMRI image is measuring the hemodynamic activity with high spatial resolution, and it can be seen as an indirect measurement of neuronal activity.

It is interesting and fantastic that we can see that the brain is thinking.

Maybe it is good that we cannot see what we are thinking of.

At least not yet.

Reference List, Chapter 10

1 Collaboration between Bengt Långström and Bengt Nielsen. With permission of Bengt L.
2 Collaboration between Bengt Långström and Bengt Nielsen. With permission of Bengt L.
3 Principle of the Gamma Camera: With courtesy: Imaging and Radioanalytical Techniques in Interdisciplinary Research—Fundamentals and Cutting Edge Applications, by Faycal Kharfi. © 2013 The Author(s). Licensee IntechOpen. This chapter is distributed under the terms of the Creative Commons Attribution 3.0 License, which permits unrestricted use, distribution, and reproduction in any medium, provided the original work is properly cited.
4 https://upload.wikimedia.org/wikipedia/commons/c/c1/PET-schema.png
5 https://en.wikipedia.org/wiki/Positron_emission_tomography#/media/File:PET-detectorsystem_2.png
6 By Nora Volkow—www.er.doe.gov/accomplishments_awards/Decades_Discovery/94.html, Public Domain,

7 https://commons.wikimedia.org/wiki/File:Viewer_medecine_nucleaire_keosys. JPG#/media/File:Viewer_medecine_nucleaire_keosys.JPG

8 https://commons.wikimedia.org/w/index.php?curid=39243250

9 Illustrations modified by Bengt Nielsen, https://en.wikipedia.org/wiki/Mammography

10 Illustrations modified by Bengt Nielsen, https://en.wikipedia.org/wiki/Breast_MRI

11 Image Courtesy Bengt Långström. Collaboration between Bengt Långström & Bengt Nielsen

12 https://en.wikipedia.org/wiki/Sensitivity_and_specificity

13 Bengt Nielsen, Own Work

14 12891 2006 Article 297 Fig3 HTML.jpg. 30-year old male patient with confirmed AS (duration inflammatory back pain 7 years)

15 SAGITTAL-FRFSE-T2 MRI.jpg. https://upload.wikimedia.org/wikipedia/commons/2/28/SAGITTAL-FRFSE-T2_MRI.jpg

11

MICROSCOPY AND OTHER MEDTECH EQUIPMENT FOR USE IN THE OPERATING ROOM

Antonie van Leeuwenhoek developed the microscope in the year 1676, and this development has had a significant impact on healthcare developments. Let's have a look at this impact and how the microscope has developed and how it has been integrated into healthcare research for both diagnosis and treatment.

Over the past three centuries, a vast number of technological developments and manufacturing breakthroughs have led to significantly advanced microscope designs featuring dramatically improved image quality.

These resolution limitations are often referred to as the diffraction barrier, which restricts the ability of optical instruments to distinguish between two objects separated by a lateral distance of less than approximately half the wavelength of light used to image the specimen.

Today, we have many different types of microscopes:

- Light/optical microscopes
- Electron microscopes:
  - Scanning electron microscopes (SEM)
  - Transmission electron microscopes (TEM)
  - Reflection electron microscopes (REM)
- X-ray microscopes
- Fluorescence microscopes
- STED microscopes

Before we discuss the principles of different types of microscopes, it is helpful to have a sense of the sizes of different objects to be looked at with different types of microscopes (Figure 11.1).

Light/optical microscopes use wavelengths between 400 nm and 800 nm (Figure 11.2).

The maximum magnification is around 80×–100×. They can be used for viewing living cells and insects, performing dissections, or assessing clinical blood and tissue.

DOI: 10.1201/9781003393320-13

What are the sizes of things in our surroundings?

nm – nanometer = 10^{-9} meter

μm – micro meter = 10^{-6} meter

mm – millimeter = 10^{-3} meter

Atom:	0.1 nm
DNA:	1 nm
Carbon nanotube:	5-10 nm
Transistor:	35 nm
Red blood cells:	10 μm

Figure 11.1   Sizes of objects for reference with different microscope capabilities.[1]

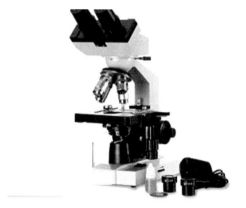

Figure 11.2   Optical/light microscope. (en.wikipedia.org)[2]

11.1   Electron Microscopes

An electron microscope (Figure 11.3) is a microscope that uses a beam of accelerated electrons as a source of illumination. As the wavelength of an electron can be up to 100,000 times shorter than that of visible light photons, electron microscopes have a higher resolving power than light microscopes and can, therefore, reveal the structure of smaller objects. A scanning transmission electron microscope (Figure 11.4) has achieved better than

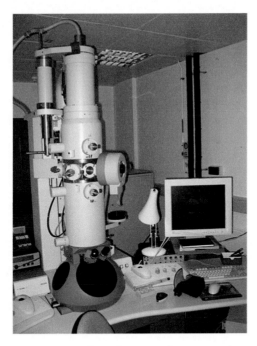

Figure 11.3   The outside look of an electron microscope. (en.wikipedia.org)[3]

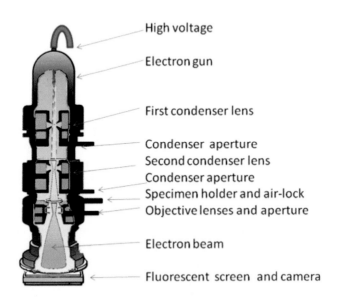

Transmission Electron Microscope

Figure 11.4   The inside of a transmission electron microscope. (en.wikipedia.org)[4]

50 picometers (50×10^{-12}) resolution and magnifications of up to about 10,000,000×, whereas most light microscopes are limited by diffraction to about 200 nanometers (200×10^{-9}) resolution and useful magnifications below 2000×.[5]

A scanning electron microscope (SEM) is a type of electron microscope that produces images of a sample by scanning the surface with a focused beam of electrons. The electrons interact with atoms in the sample, producing various signals that contain information about the surface topography and composition of the sample. The electron beam is scanned in a raster scan pattern, and the position of the beam is combined with the intensity of the detected signal to produce an image.[6]

In a reflection electron microscope (REM), as in TEM, an electron beam is incident on a surface, but instead of using the transmission (TEM) or secondary electrons (SEM), the reflected beam of elastically scattered electrons is detected. This technique is typically coupled with reflection high-energy electron diffraction (RHEED) and reflection high-energy loss spectroscopy (RHELS).[7]

An X-ray microscope uses electromagnetic radiation in the soft X-ray band to produce magnified images of objects. Since X-rays penetrate most objects, there is no need to specially prepare them for X-ray microscopy observations. Unlike visible light, X-rays do not reflect or refract easily and are invisible to the human eye. Therefore, an X-ray microscope exposes the film or uses a charge-coupled device (CCD) detector to detect X-rays that pass through the specimen. It is a contrast imaging technology using the difference in absorption of soft X-rays in the water window region (wavelengths: 2.34–4.4 nm, energies: 280–530 eV) by the carbon atom (main element composing the living cell) and the oxygen atom (an element of water).[8]

Fluorescence microscopy is an imaging technique used in light microscopes that allows the excitation of fluorophores and subsequent detection of the fluorescence signal. Fluorescence is produced when light excites or moves an electron to a higher energy state, immediately generating light of a longer wavelength, lower energy, and different color to the original light absorbed.

To visualize labeled molecules in the sample, fluorescence microscopes require a very powerful light source and a dichroic mirror to reflect light at the desired excitation/emission wavelength. The filtered excitation light then passes through the objective to be focused onto the sample, and the emitted light is filtered back onto the detector for image digitalization.[9]

STED microscopy is one of several types of super-resolution microscopy techniques that have recently been developed to bypass the diffraction limit of light microscopy to increase resolution.

STED stands for stimulated emission depletion microscopy.

STED is a deterministic functional technique that exploits the non-linear response of fluorophores commonly used to label biological samples in order to achieve an improvement in resolution.

STED microscopy allows for images to be taken at resolutions below the diffraction limit.

The STED technique was developed by Stefan Hell and Jan Wichmann in 1994, and was first experimentally demonstrated by Hell and Thomas Klar in 1999. Hell was awarded the Nobel Prize in Chemistry in 2014 for its development.[10]

The time between diagnosis and therapy is becoming shorter, and the physical distance between the two is also becoming shorter (Figure 11.5).

Can they be fully integrated?

Diagnostic tools are key and come first, but fixing/curing the patient is the most important goal for our healthcare organizations.

The time between diagnosis and treatment must be kept as short as possible in order to avoid the disease from spreading or becoming worse. The time between diagnosis and treatment is important for most diseases, cancers, heart diseases, and neurological diseases.

Today, there is a physical distance between the diagnostic department and the place where the treatment will happen. This also means that often, there will be a considerable time between diagnosis and therapy. In many situations, this is an unwanted and negative effect.

Let's look at a few examples:

A patient comes into a hospital with a suspected problem with his/her thyroid gland. The patient will then most likely be going through a SPECT exam with an iodine tracer injected and a gamma camera investigation. If the problem is cancer, then depending on the stage of cancer, the treatment could very well be a targeted treatment with iodine 131 (^{131}I).

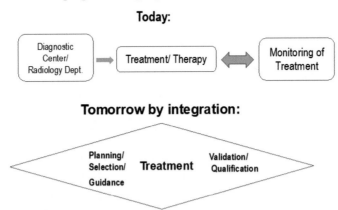

Figure 11.5 An idea of how diagnosis and therapy might be combined in the future. (Bengt Nielsen, own illustration.)[11]

Radioactive iodine can be a targeted treatment in the case of thyroid cancer. The radioactive iodine circulates throughout your body in your bloodstream, but it is mainly taken up by thyroid cells, having little effect on other cells in your body. Thyroid cancer cells in your body pick up the iodine. The radiation in the iodine then kills the cancer cells.

It is only suitable for some types of thyroid cancer. It is a treatment for the following:

- Follicular thyroid cancer (the follicular phase is the longest step in the menstrual cycle, lasting from the first day of a period to ovulation, meaning the release of the egg).
- Papillary thyroid cancer (the most common form of well-differentiated thyroid cancer).

It can treat the cancer even if it has spread. But even if you have one of these types of thyroid cancers, this treatment may not be necessary or suitable for you. Not all cancer cells take up iodine, so you may have a test dose to see if they do take up iodine.

11.2   The Hybrid Operating Room

A hybrid operating room is an advanced procedural space that combines a traditional operating room with an image-guided interventional suite (Figure 11.6). This combination allows for highly complex, advanced surgical procedures. Many different modalities and technical solutions are being tested and evaluated.

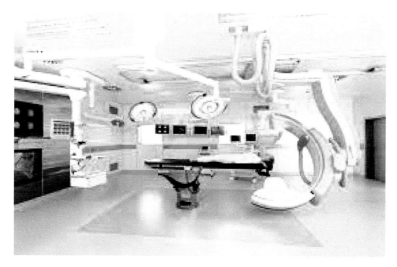

Figure 11.6   An example of a hybrid operation suite. The operating table is surrounded by different imaging equipment that can be used before, during, and after the surgery.

The coupling of diagnosis and therapy is giving improved conditions for challenging surgeries. As an example, many feature versatile imaging equipment, such as robot-assisted angiography systems, which allow physicians to perform 3D image reconstructions in real time during a procedure. Another more typical example is the catheter-assisted heart valve replacement, which was introduced in Europe just a decade ago—several thousand patients underwent transcatheter aortic valve replacement therapy in Europe between 2007 and 2011 alone.

11.3   Diagnostic Tools in the Operating Theater

In connection with cancer surgery, it is a great advantage if the surgeon can get immediate response/knowledge if he has managed to cut out all the whole cancerous tissue. Today, there are techniques available where it is possible to inject a dye and, via a stimulating laser, see if the dye binding to the tissue gives an indication if there are cancer cells still in the area around what has been removed. The technique is called fluorescence analysis or fluorescence spectroscopy.

Another way is to bring diagnostic tools into or adjacent to the operating room (Figures 11.7 and 11.8). It can be standard diagnostic tools, like an ultrasound, X-rays of different kinds, gamma camera, CT, and MRI.

There are also very technically advanced solutions with the possibility to seamlessly move the patient back and forth between a diagnostic unit and the operating table. The diagnostics could be as follows: MRI, CT, or any type of diagnostic equipment.

The mass spectroscopy pen collects biological molecules from a tissue sample surface via a solid-liquid extraction mechanism and transports the molecules to a mass spectrometer for analysis (Figure 11.9). The composition

Ultrasound equipment that can be used in an operating room

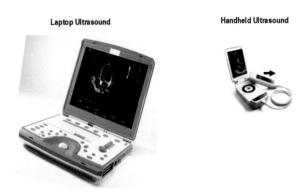

Laptop Ultrasound

Handheld Ultrasound

Figure 11.7   Ultrasound equipment suitable for use in an operating suite. One ultrasound unit is like a portable computer (left), and another is a handheld unit (right).

PET-imaging with approximately 1 mm spatial resolution

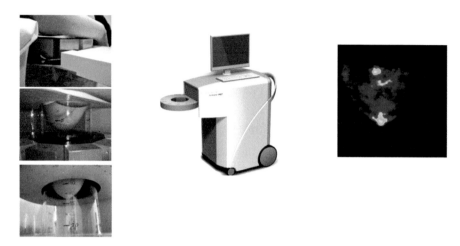

Figure 11.8   Mobile PET capable of being placed in an operating room. Spatial resolution is down to 1 mm. (Image courtesy of Jose-Maria Benloch Baviera.)[12]

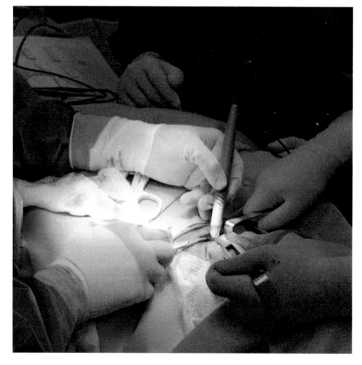

Figure 11.9   Mass spectrometer used for cancer identification during an operation. (en.wikipedia.org; Image courtesy of MS-Pen)[13]

of the extracted molecules can then be used to predict if the tissue sample analyzed contains cancerous cells using machine learning algorithms and statistical models.

This technology has the potential to support surgeons in removing a tumor and leaving far fewer cancerous tissue and, as a consequence, avoid or minimize the risk for the cancer to reoccur after the surgery.

11.4   Integration of Different Technologies

Simultaneous intervention, intravascular ultrasound, and measurement of blood pressure inside the vessels

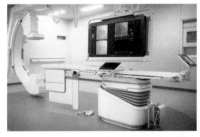
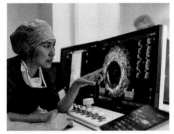

Diagnostics and treatment in the same session.

Figure 11.10   Simultaneous intravascular ultrasound and blood pressure measurement inside a blood vessel.

11.5   Ultrasound and Focused Ultrasound for Diagnosis and Treatment

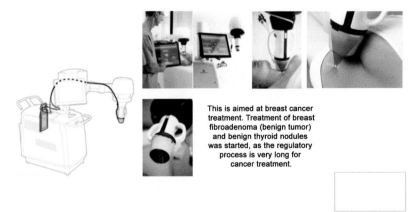

This is aimed at breast cancer treatment. Treatment of breast fibroadenoma (benign tumor) and benign thyroid nodules was started, as the regulatory process is very long for cancer treatment.

Figure 11.11   A technique where ultrasound is used for diagnosis, followed by focused ultrasound before treatment. The example shows testing the treatment of breast fibroadenoma and benign thyroid nodules. Starting with benign validations is due to the very long regulatory process for cancer treatment.

11.6   MR-Guided Focused Ultrasound

The principle of MR-guided focused ultrasound (FUS) (Figures 11.12, 11.13, and 11.14) is the same as the ultrasound-guided FUS with the difference that, now, the imaging modality is MRI. With the excellent soft tissue contrast of MRI, it is possible to follow the treatment continuously while the treatment is in progress.

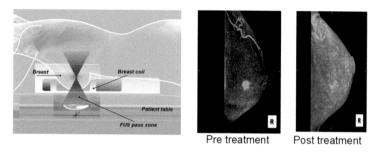

MR-Guided Focused Ultrasound (MRgFUS)
Breast Cancer Phase III Study
(97% average tumor removal)

Pre treatment   Post treatment

When waves are concentrated, they
produce heat only at the focus.

Figure 11.12   Principle of MR-guided focused ultrasound. The example shows the treatment of breast cancer. (Image courtesy of Insightec.)[14]

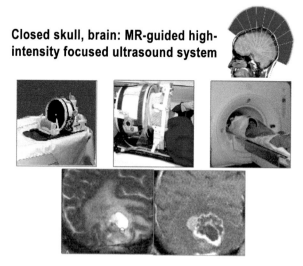

Closed skull, brain: MR-guided high-intensity focused ultrasound system

Figure 11.13   MR-guided focused ultrasound (MRgFUS) for brain lesions. (Image courtesy of Insightec.)[15]

MR Surgical Suite: Focused Ultrasound

Tumor Ablation
MR: Real-time thermal feedback
and monitoring
FUS: Non-invasive, localized
tumor ablation

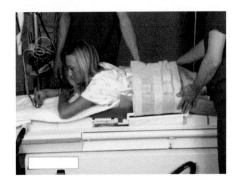

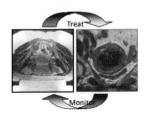

Figure 11.14   MR-guided high-intensity focused ultrasound system: Kidney and uterine treatment. (Image courtesy of Insightec.)[16]

The treatment unit is inserted into the MRI magnet tunnel, and the treatment can then be followed live, and the outcome can be seen while the treatment is in progress.

11.7   Diagnostic and Treatment Equipment Designed for Potential Use at Smaller Clinics

Laparoscopy is a type of surgical procedure that allows a surgeon to access the inside of the abdomen and pelvis without having to make large incisions on the skin (Figure 11.15). This procedure is also known as keyhole surgery or minimally invasive surgery.

11.8   Future Integration of Diagnosis and Therapy

Research tools are rapidly moving into clinical tests and validation and, finally, into clinical practice.

There are ongoing research ideas and projects that could materialize in the future.

Some examples are as follows.

11.8.1   MR-Linac

The MR is integrated with a Linac (a linear accelerator device that can accelerate charged elementary particles to a very high energy level) (Figure 11.16).

These accelerated charged particles can then be used to treat, for instance, cancer. Normally, a CT is used for treatment planning. In this case, the same type of radiation is used both for diagnosis and for treatment.

Ultrasound and high-intensity focused ultrasound, laparscopy treatement

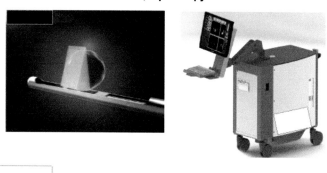

Figure 11.15   Ultrasound and high-intensity focused ultrasound for laparoscopy treatment of thyroid nodules.

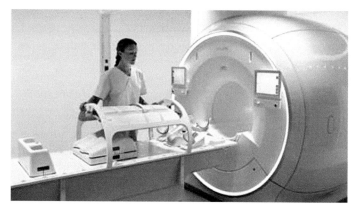

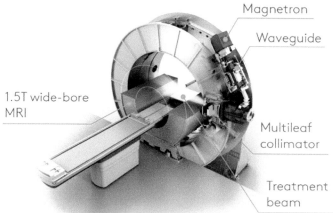

Magnetron

Waveguide

1.5T wide-bore MRI

Multileaf collimator

Treatment beam

Figure 11.16   The MR-Linac principle of operation.

This means that the attenuation coefficient can be calculated rather simply and robustly. Using the MR for planning means that there need to be some difficult approximations, as the MR image is based on very different physics, and hence, the attenuation correction is a limitation. Strategies for the development of approximative corrections that can be said to be good enough are ongoing.

The MR-Linac is the first of its kind to combine radiotherapy with real-time MR imaging, giving a real-time follow-up of the progress of the treatment. For the moment, this new tool is under clinical validation on a few sites in the world. The only thing we can say today is that it is a very interesting and certainly promising opportunity. This would certainly become a game changer when it comes to cancer treatment. Let's follow this carefully. Soon, we will know the outcome.

11.8.2 Endoscopy

The endoscope can be moved inside the intestinal system with the guidance of an X-ray system (Figure 11.17).

The endoscope is equipped with a unit for ablation, and this can be used to remove polyps that potentially could develop into cancer in the intestinal system at a later stage. The polyps can be removed directly during the diagnostic session.

In Figure 11.17b, you can see why early diagnosis is so important. The small polyps that can be removed with the endoscope have not grown to the size where they can start to spread to the lymph nodes.

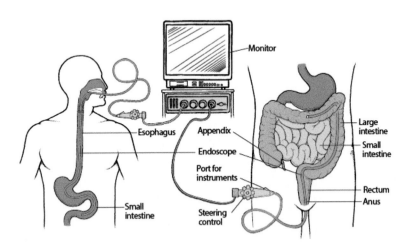

Figure 11.17a Endoscopy tube that, after insertion via the rectum, can diagnose and use ablation to take away polyps that could develop into cancer at a later stage. The endoscope can be navigated through the intestinal system with the help of fluoroscopy (real-time X-ray method discussed earlier). (Illustration courtesy of Colorectal Cancer Alliance.)[17]

Cancer progression - early detection is key

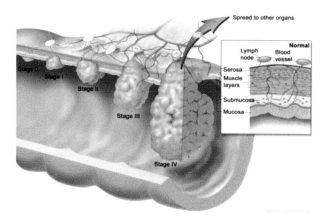

Figure 11.17b

11.8.3   *Taking Endoscopy into a New Reality*

One company has developed a unique system with the capability of doing high-resolution microscopy via an endoscopy, giving detailed information about tissues without having to take out samples to analyze on a stand-alone microscope (Figures 11.18 and 11.19).

11.9   Stereotactic Magnetic Navigation System for High-Precision Catheterization and Ablations

Stereotactic magnetic navigation systems (Figure 11.20) can deliver very high-precision ablations: For example, in the heart, for atrial fibrillations and other diseases, where you need very high precision.

Many instruments are already installed in cardiological clinics.

11.10   Magnetoencephalography

Magnetoencephalography (MEG) is an instrument able to measure the magnetic field activity coming from the nerve cells in the brain. The MEG instrument can be found in specialized clinics and hospitals aimed at research as well as some clinical applications, like epilepsy and dementia. Sometimes, the technique is also used as a preparatory tool before brain surgery.

The MEG measures the very tiny magnetic fields erected when brain cells are activated. Special attention has been directed toward Parkinson's disease (PD) recently in some research projects. The registration is rather long, approximately four hours.

Real-Time Optical Biopsy

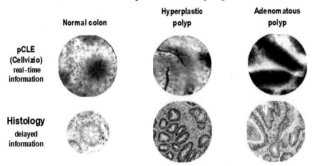

Figure 11.18   Real-time optical biopsy diagram.

Endoscopy + Microscopy In Vivo

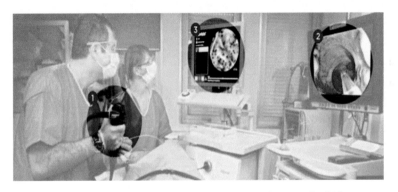

Figure 11.19   Illustration showing the setup for real-time optical biopsy.

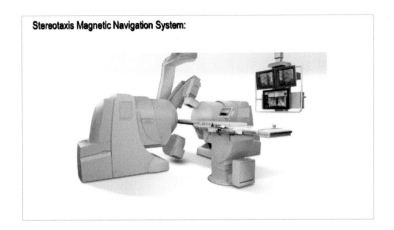

Figure 11.20   Stereotaxis magnetic navigation system.

Reference List, Chapter 11

1 Table by Bengt Nielsen: Sizes of Objects for Reference to Different Microscopes Capabilities. Data from en.wikipedia.org.
2 https://en.wikipedia.org/wiki/Optical_microscope
3 https://en.wikipedia.org/wiki/Electron_microscope
4 https://en.wikipedia.org/wiki/Transmission_electron_microscopy
5 Description Electron Microscope
6 Description Scanning Electron Microscope
7 Description Reflection Electron Microscope
8 Description X-ray Microscope
9 Description Fluorescence Microscope
10 Description STED Microscope
11 Bengt Nielsen, Own Work
12 Image courtesy of Jose-Maria Benloch Baviera, Mobile PET for operating suite
13 https://en.wikipedia.org/wiki/MasSpec_Pen
14 Image Courtesy of Insightec, MR Guided Focused Ultrasound, Breast Cancer Treatment
15 Image Courtesy of Insightec, MR Guided Ultrasound, Treatment of Brain Lesions
16 Image Courtesy of Insightec, MR Guided Ultrasound, Kidney and Uterine Treatment
17 Image Courtesy of Colorectal Cancer Alliance

Part 3

PRESENT TIME

12

DEVELOPMENTS AND DISCOVERIES IN THE 21ST CENTURY TO THE PRESENT (2022)

12.1 Artificial Organs

1. *Eyes*: Skin cells from individuals with rare genetic diseases are being used to grow eyecups. This will help scientists isolate disease-causing genes and develop targeted treatments for patients.
2. *Heart*: Pluripotent stem cells (cells that can become several types of cells) are being used to form tissue resembling that of a human heart. In one instance, this tissue started to beat when it was given an electric shock. Exciting development!
3. *Skin*: Doctors in the United States have developed a way to treat severe burns. By using a thin layer of stem cells taken from the actual patient, they spray them onto the wound, which allows the skin to heal evenly and completely. These skin cells are duplicated in the lab before being sprayed onto the patient. This process alleviates the need for painful skin grafts that are very prone to developing serious infections.
4. *Bone*: Stem cells taken from bone marrow are suspended in a collagen gel and then exposed to nano vibrations. This creates a putty-like substance used to graft bones back together. This putty is typically softer than our bones, but it has been used successfully to heal big bones, making them harder and stronger than before the break.
5. *Muscles*: Bundles of muscles are being grown that twitch and respond to electrical stimuli. These muscles are grown from pluripotent stem cells taken from biopsies. Lab-grown muscles can be used in the development of new drugs needed to treat muscle conditions and to test the efficiency of treatments prior to drug use in humans.
6. *Brains*: Scientists are using stem cells from children's milk teeth and reprogramming them into neurons. These organoids closely resemble the early embryonic stages of the brain. The information gathered from this study helps scientists study the genetic mutations that take place in the brain.
7. *Liver*: Using stem cells, scientists have grown liver cells that, when transplanted into mice, have actually formed their own blood supply and matured into adult liver cells. When tested, these livers showed some normal liver functions. Hopes are that, eventually, doctors can transplant fully functioning lab-grown livers in humans.

DOI: 10.1201/9781003393320-15

8. *HIV or AIDS treatments* have come a long way since the inception of the disease in the 1980s. Originally, treatment consisted of a single regimen that was ineffective because there were many medications taken individually. It was hard for patients to stay on schedule taking so many medications, and the side effects were numerous.

9. *Monotherapies* (single-drug treatments) also allowed HIV to change or mutate into a form that eventually stopped responding to the individual drugs. In other words, the disease was becoming immune to the treatments available.

10. In 2006, the FDA approved *Atripla,* which combined three antiretroviral drugs into one, which improved the treatment for AIDS. With three drugs being compiled into one, it was easier to stay on schedule, and the side effects were decreased.

11. *Stribild,* a medication approved for HIV patients in 2013 combined four HIV antiretroviral medications into one dose, which was even more effective in controlling the symptoms for these patients.

In November 2017, a big breakthrough in treating HIV came through. According to the FDA, Juluca was approved and was the first two-drug single-dose treatment for AIDS patients that were already on an antiretroviral treatment regimen.

This was great for those patients, but patients that were not on an antiretroviral treatment already were still out of luck. In April 2019, Dovato, a two-drug single-dose treatment for HIV was approved for people who have not been on antiretroviral therapy. This breakthrough now makes it possible for all HIV patients to be on effective single-dose therapy.

12.2   Control of Heart Disease

Thanks to advancements in the area of cardiovascular health, deaths due to heart disease have dropped significantly over the past ten years. If attended quickly, a person having a heart attack can be successfully treated by busting the blockage that prevents the blood from circulating with t-PA, a genetically engineered tissue plasminogen activator. Plaque in the blood vessels can then be opened by inserting a stent, which is put into the artery. The damaged artery is then replaced with a new vessel through a procedure referred to as bypass surgery. These advancements have dramatically increased the survival rate of heart disease patients.

12.3   Targeted Therapy in Cancer Treatment

Until recently, surgery, chemotherapy, and radiation therapy were the only choices for treating cancer patients. These therapies not only attack cancerous cells, but they also attack healthy cells, which causes a new set of problems. When given the option of these types of treatments, the chance of killing cancer usually outweighs the result of having cancer, so the side effects are expected and are dealt with as they come.

Within the past 10 years, targeted cancer therapies have been developed that work in one of two ways:

1. Interfere with the spread of cancer by blocking the cells that are involved in the tumor growth.
2. Identify and kill the deadly cancer cells.

Either way, they target the cancerous cells and attack them but leave the healthy cells alone. Researchers are focusing their energy on targeted therapies, and more than 25 drugs have been approved by the FDA for this purpose.

These targeted therapy drugs will allow treatments to be individualized based on tumor molecular makeup. This type of treatment does away with the side effects caused by chemo and radiation, which is great news for those affected by this disease.

12.3.1   The Gamma Knife

A Gamma Knife (also known as the Leksell Gamma Knife) is used to treat brain tumors by administering high-intensity gamma radiation therapy in a manner that concentrates the radiation over a small volume. The device was invented in 1967 at the Karolinska Institute in Stockholm, Sweden, by Lars Leksell, Romanian-born neurosurgeon Ladislau Steiner, and radiobiologist Börje Larsson from Uppsala University, Sweden. The first Gamma Knife was brought to the United States through an arrangement between US neurosurgeon Robert Wheeler Rand and Leksell and was given to the University of California, Los Angeles (UCLA), in 1979.

A Gamma Knife typically contains 201 cobalt-60 sources of approximately 30 curies each (1 TBq = terabecquerel) placed in a hemispheric array in a heavily shielded assembly.

The device aims gamma radiation through a target point in the patient's brain. The patient wears a specialized helmet that is surgically fixed to the skull so that the brain tumor remains stationary at the target point of the gamma rays.

An ablative dose of radiation is thereby sent through the tumor in one treatment session while surrounding brain tissues are relatively spared.

Gamma Knife therapy, like all radiosurgery, uses doses of radiation to kill cancer cells and shrink tumors, delivered precisely to avoid damaging healthy brain tissue. Gamma Knife radiosurgery can accurately focus many beams of gamma radiation on one or more tumors.

Each individual beam is of relatively low intensity, so the radiation has little effect on intervening brain tissue and is concentrated only at the tumor itself.

Gamma Knife radiosurgery has proven effective for patients with benign or malignant brain tumors up to 4 cm (1.6 in) in size and vascular malformations, such as arteriovenous malformation (AVM), pain, and other functional problems. This can also be used for the treatment of trigeminal neuralgia. The procedure may be used repeatedly on the patients. Trigeminal neuralgia is a condition characterized by pain coming from the trigeminal nerve, which starts near the top of the ear and splits in three, toward the eye, cheek, and jaw.

The Leksell Gamma Knife (Figure 12.1) consists of around 200 small radioactive radiation sources that are arranged in the helmet of the unit. The small radioactive sources are all pointing to a specific point in space with the aim to irradiate the cancer cells. By spreading out the radioactive sources over the helmet, the negative effect of the radiation on the healthy brain tissues are avoided. However, the radiation dose to the single point where the rays meet is very high. The radioactive sources are ^{60}Co, cobalt-60. This instrument has been very successful in treating brain tumors with high precision and avoiding harm to healthy tissues.

12.3.2   Proton Therapy

In the field of medical treatment, proton beam therapy, or proton radiotherapy, is a type of particle therapy that uses a beam of protons to irradiate diseased tissue, most often to treat cancer. The main advantage of proton therapy over other types of external beam radiotherapy (e.g., photon

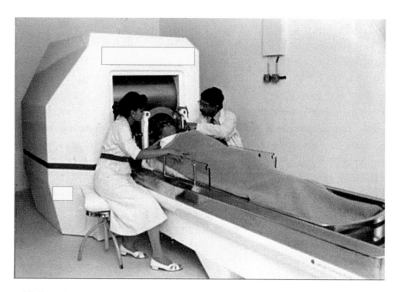

Figure 12.1   The Leksell Gamma Knife is an apparatus that irradiates and kills cancer cells in the human brain.

radiation therapy) is that the dose of protons is deposited over a narrow range of depth, which results in minimal entry, exit, or scattered radiation dose to healthy nearby tissues.

When evaluating whether to treat a tumor with photon (linear accelerator) or proton therapy, physicians may choose proton therapy if it is important to deliver a higher radiation dose to targeted tissues while significantly decreasing radiation to nearby organs at risk.

The Model Policy for Proton Beam Therapy states that proton therapy is considered reasonable in instances were sparing the surrounding normal tissue "cannot be adequately achieved with photon-based radiotherapy" and can benefit the patient. Like photon radiation therapy, proton therapy is often used in conjunction with surgery and/or chemotherapy to treat cancer most effectively.

The phenomenon of the Bragg peak of ejected protons gives proton therapy advantages over other forms of radiation since most of the proton's energy is deposited within a limited distance, so tissue beyond this range (and to some extent also, tissue inside this range) is spared from the effects of radiation.

This property of protons, which has been called the depth charge effect by allowing for conformal dose distributions to be created around even very irregularly shaped targets and for higher doses to targets surrounded or backstopped by radiation-sensitive structures, such as the optic chiasm or brainstem. There is today a growing number of proton therapy units around the world. They are used to treat cancers in critical parts of the body where the radiation beams may hurt healthy and radiation-sensitive tissue. It should be noted that the treatment plan will be more exact; using protons as the dose delivery is more precise compared to photons, as the dose can be higher and still avoid hitting sensitive tissues being close to the target.[1]

12.4   Nanomedicine

Nanomedicine is the medical application of nanotechnology. Nanomedicine ranges from the medical applications of nanomaterials and biological devices to nano-electronic biosensors and even possible future applications of molecular nanotechnology, such as biological machines (for instance, mimicking what is happening within a cell). Current problems for nanomedicine involve understanding the issues related to toxicity and environmental impact of nanoscale materials (materials whose structure is of the scale of nanometers).

The application of nanotechnology in medicine is an innovative use of nanomaterials. These tiny, nano biosensors and nanoparticles make it possible to perform a corrective procedure right in the affected molecules. This is a real and extremely targeted therapy. Progress in this area has been quick, with almost 130 drugs developed around the world.

When using nanomedicine, it is possible to target areas of infection or diseased areas without harming the surrounding tissue. Many new targeted techniques for diagnosis and therapy are based on nanomaterials, and it is an expanding part of medicine today.

12.4.1 Definition

According to the EC recommendation, nanomaterial refers to a natural, incidental, or manufactured material comprising particles, either in an unbound state or as an aggregate wherein one or more external dimensions are in the size range of 1–100 nm for ≥ 50% of the particles, according to the number size distribution. In cases of environment, health, safety, or competitiveness concerns, the number size distribution threshold of 50% may be substituted by a threshold between 1% and 50%.

12.4.2 Size

The most important feature to consider is size because it is applicable to a huge range of materials. The conventional range is from 1 to 100 nm. However, there is no evidence of a limit to an exact size. The maximum size that a material can have to be considered nanomaterial is an arbitrary value because the psychochemical and biological characteristics of the materials do not change abruptly at 100 nm.[2]

12.5   3D-Printed Body Parts

Originating at the turn of the 21st century, it was found that living cells could be sprayed through inkjet printers without being harmed in any way.

Today, different cell types are combined with polymers and sprayed through various printheads. According to *Reader's Digest*, the polymers help the cell structure keep its shape, making it possible to spray layers upon layers that bind together and grow into living, functional tissues.

The body parts that have been successfully printed include the following:

- Bionic eye
- Antibacterial tooth
- Heart
- Skin
- Bionic ear
- Elastic bone
- Ovary

Scientists have taken printed muscles and ears and planted them into animals, which unified with their hosts. They have implanted printed ovaries into mice who conceived and gave birth with these artificial organs. It is exciting to think of the possibilities that 3D printing can offer for humans.[3]

12.6   Laparoscopic Surgery

Laparoscopic surgery has become as much of a normal procedure as conventional surgery. This minimally invasive surgery is done through one or more small incisions using small tubes and tiny cameras and instruments.

The benefits of laparoscopic surgery include the following:

- Less pain
- Shorter hospital stays
- Fewer complications
- Smaller scars
- Shorter recovery time

Although this procedure was developed in the 1980s, it wasn't until the 21st century that it was perfected and began being used in many surgery procedures.

The use of laparoscopic surgery has opened the door to minimally invasive surgeries, allowing patients that might not be able to withstand a conventional procedure the opportunity to obtain a cure.[4]

12.7   New Class of Antibiotics

We are facing a major global health threat with the large increase in bacterial resistance against our current antibiotics. It has been 30 years since a new class of antibiotics has been discovered. As we grow and evolve, we tend to develop a resistance to what we have been given over the years.

Teixobactin is a new class of antibiotics that is being developed to combat multidrug-resistant bacterial pathogens that are currently being used.

Teixobactin is a natural compound that can help us wipe out the superbugs that are invading our culture. Scientists are making great progress toward developing a version of teixobactin that can be prescribed to humans. They are hopeful that this new class of antibiotics will aid in killing serious infections, such as septicemia and tuberculosis.[5]

12.8   The Human Genome Project Draft: June 2000

The Human Genome Project (HGP) was an international scientific research project with the goal of determining the base pairs that make up human DNA and of identifying, mapping, and sequencing all the genes of the human genome from both a physical and a functional standpoint. It remains the world's largest collaborative biological project. Planning started after the idea was picked up in 1984 by the US government; the project formally launched in 1990 and was declared essentially complete on April 14, 2003, but included only about 85% of the genome.

The level of complete genome was achieved in May 2021, with a remainder of only 0.3% bases covered by potential issues. The missing Y chromosome was added in January 2022.

Funding came from the American government through the National Institutes of Health (NIH) as well as numerous other groups from around the world. A parallel project was conducted outside the government by the Celera Corporation, or Celera Genomics, which was formally launched in 1998.

Most of the government-sponsored sequencing was performed in 20 universities and research centers in the United States, the United Kingdom, Japan, France, Germany, and China.

12.8.1   Completion of the Human Genome Project

The human genome is all the genes that make up our DNA. In 2013, scientists completed the first-ever draft that sequenced the human genome.

Information from DNA is used to develop new ways to treat, cure, or even prevent thousands of diseases affecting mankind.

Gene sequencing has already helped researchers identify single genes that cause diseases, enabling them to create treatments. This gene therapy is a huge step toward biomedical advancements and personalized healthcare.

The hope held by the medical community and the public is that the human genome draft sequencing will allow scientists and researchers to develop treatments or even cures for all diseases.[6]

12.9   The First Remote Surgery or Telesurgery Was Performed: 2001

Remote surgery is the ability of a doctor to perform surgery on a patient even though they are not physically at the same location. It is a form of telepresence. A robot surgical system generally consists of one or more arms (controlled by the surgeon), a master controller (console), and a sensory system giving feedback to the user. Remote surgery combines elements of robotics; telecommunication, such as high-speed data connections; and elements of management information systems. While the field of robotic surgery is rather well established, most of these robots are controlled by surgeons at the location of the surgery. Remote surgery is remote work for surgeons, where the physical distance between the surgeon and the patient is less relevant. It promises to allow the expertise of specialized surgeons to be available to patients worldwide, without the need for patients to travel beyond their local hospital.[7]

12.10   Alert to WHO on the Threat of the SARS Virus, Triggering the Most Effective Response to an Epidemic in History: 2003

Severe acute respiratory syndrome (SARS) is the first severe and readily transmissible new disease to emerge in the 21st century. Initially recognized as a global threat in mid-March 2003, SARS was successfully contained in less than four months, largely because of an unprecedented level of international collaboration and cooperation.

The SARS outbreak has also shown how, in a closely interconnected and interdependent world, a new and poorly understood infectious disease can have an adverse effect not only on public health but also on economic growth, trade, tourism, business and industrial performance, and political and social stability.[8]

12.11   The First Partial Face Transplant: 2005

In 2005, surgeons gave a French woman, Isabelle Dinoire, a new nose and mouth after she was attacked and bitten by her pet dog.

She told the BBC in 2009 that when she looked in the mirror, she saw a mixture of herself and the donor. "The donor is always with me," she said.[9]

12.12   HPV Vaccine Approved: 2006

Human papillomavirus (HPV) is a common virus that can cause cancers later in life. The first vaccine against cervical cancer has been fast-tracked to approval by US drug regulators. The disease kills 233,000 women worldwide each year.

The Food and Drug Administration approved the sale of Gardasil, produced by the US pharmaceutical firm Merck, after a six-month fast-track clinical test. The vaccine protects against HPV, which causes genital warts that can lead to cancer. HPV infections are responsible for 70% of cervical cancer, which is the second most common cancer among women worldwide. The vaccine is effective against four key types of the virus.[10]

12.13   The Second Improved Rotavirus Vaccine Approved: 2006

Infection with rotavirus is a leading cause of severe diarrhea in infants and young children in the United States and worldwide. In the United States, the disease occurs more often during the winter, with the most activity occurring from November to May. Most children, whether in the United States or elsewhere, are infected with rotavirus before they are two years old.[11]

12.14   The Visual Prosthetic (Bionic Eye) Argus II: 2007

Argus retinal prosthesis, also known as a bionic eye, is an electronic retinal implant manufactured by the American company Second Sight Medical Products. It is used as a visual prosthesis to improve the vision of people with severe cases of retinitis pigmentosa, a genetic disorder of the eyes that causes loss of vison.

The Argus II version of the system was approved for marketing in the European Union in March 2011, and it received approval in the United States in February 2013 under a humanitarian device exemption. The Argus II system costs about US$150,000, excluding the cost of implantation surgery and training to learn to use the device.[12]

12.15 First Full-Face Transplant: 2010

On March 20, 2010, a team of 30 Spanish doctors led by plastic surgeon Joan Pere Barret at the Vall d'Hebron University Hospital in Barcelona carried out the first full-face transplant on a man injured in a shooting accident. It became the first full-face transplant in the world.[13]

12.16 First Successful Uterus Transplant from a Deceased Donor: 2011

In 2011, a team in Turkey was the first to transplant a uterus from a deceased donor, but the procedure did not lead to a live birth. Ejzenberg says that attempt inspired him to begin a program in Brazil. He traveled to Sweden to learn from doctors there who have the most experience with uterine transplantation.[14]

12.17 The First Kidney Was Grown In Vitro: 2013

Scientists have implanted a laboratory-grown kidney into a rat for the first time, a medical milestone that they hope will soon lead to similar solutions for human beings needing full organ transplants. "It's the first one ever that's been implanted into an animal," said Harald Ott, MD and PhD, at the Massachusetts General Hospital Center for Regenerative Medicine and the lead researcher behind the project.[15]

12.18 The First Human Liver Was Grown from Stem Cells: 2013

Tiny functioning human livers have been grown from stem cells in the laboratory by scientists in Japan.

They said they were astounded when liver buds, the earliest stage of the organ's development, formed spontaneously.

The team, reporting their findings in *Nature*, hopes that transplanting thousands of liver buds could reverse liver failure.[16]

12.19 A 3D Printer Is Used for the First-Ever Skull Transplant: 2014

Doctors at Utrecht Medical Center in the Netherlands used a 3D printer to build a plastic prosthetic bone for what they said was the first full-skull transplant, *Dutch News* reports. The surgery was performed in December, lasting 23 hours.[17]

12.20 The First-Ever Artificial Pancreas Was Created: 2016

Based on the results of the trial, in September 2016, the FDA announced that it approved the device for use in people 14 years of age and older with type 1 diabetes—the first commercial hybrid artificial pancreas to be FDA approved (January 24, 2017).[18]

12.21   3D-Printed Heart from Human Patient's Cells: 2019

Researchers have 3D printed a heart using a patient's cells, providing hope that the technique could be used to heal hearts or engineer new ones for transplants.

"This is the first time anyone anywhere has successfully engineered and printed an entire heart replete with cells, blood vessels, ventricles and chambers," Professor Tal Dvir of Tel Aviv University's School of Molecular Cell Biology and Biotechnology said in a statement.

Professor Tal Dvir is the senior author of the research published in the journal *Advanced Science*.[19]

Reference List, Chapter 12

1 https://en.wikipedia.org/wiki/Proton_therapy
2 https://en.wikipedia.org/wiki/Nanomedicine
3 3D printed Body Parts
4 https://en.wikipedia.org/wiki/Laparoscopy
5 www.ncbi.nlm.nih.gov/pmc/articles/PMC3085877/
6 www.genome.gov/human-genome-project
7 https://en.wikipedia.org/wiki/Remote_surgery
8 www.ncbi.nlm.nih.gov/books/NBK92476/
9 https://en.wikipedia.org/wiki/Isabelle_Dinoire
10 https://pubmed.ncbi.nlm.nih.gov/17010274/
11 www.ncbi.nlm.nih.gov/pmc/articles/PMC8482027/
12 https://en.wikipedia.org/wiki/Argus_retinal_prosthesis
13 https://pubmed.ncbi.nlm.nih.gov/21772126/
14 www.scientificamerican.com/article/first-successful-uterus-transplant-from-deceased-donor-leads-to-healthy-baby/
15 www.ncbi.nlm.nih.gov/pmc/articles/PMC3989688/
16 https://www.ncbi.nlm.nih.gov/pmc/articles/PMC8402319/
17 www.nbcnews.com/science/science-news/medical-first-3-d-printed-skull-successfully-implanted-woman-n65576
18 www.niddk.nih.gov/news/archive/2017/story-discovery-artificial-pancreas-managing-type1-diabetes
19 www.ncbi.nlm.nih.gov/pmc/articles/PMC8119699/

13

OTHER IMPORTANT MEDTECH EQUIPMENT IN OUR HOSPITALS, CLINICS, AND OUTPATIENT CENTERS THAT ARE INDISPENSABLE TODAY

13.1 Blood Pressure Measurement

13.1.1 ECG Equipment

The basic principle of the electrocardiogram (ECG) is that the stimulation of a muscle alters the electrical potential of muscle fibers (Figures 13.3, 13.4, and 13.5). Cardiac cells, unlike other cells, have a property known as automaticity, which is the capacity to spontaneously initiate impulses.

There are three main components of an ECG (Figure 13.6): the P wave, which represents the depolarization of the atria; the QRS complex, which represents the depolarization of the ventricles; and the T wave, which represents the repolarization of the ventricles.

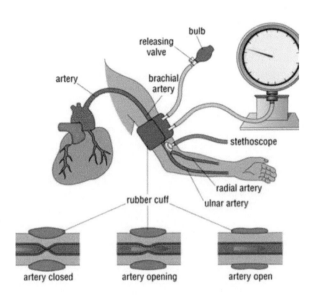

Figure 13.1 The principle of blood pressure measurement.

DOI: 10.1201/9781003393320-16

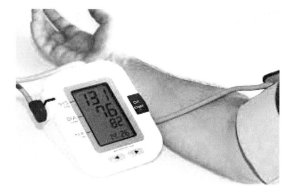

Figure 13.2   Typical commercial blood pressure unit.

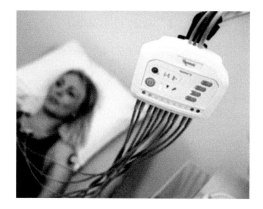

Figure 13.3   Stationary ECG unit, 12 channels.

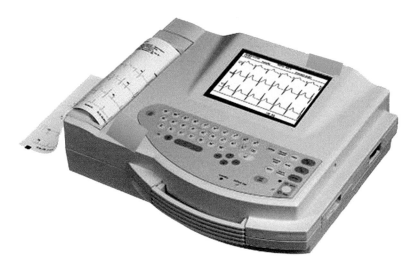

Figure 13.4   Mobile 12 channel ECG apparatus. ECG cables not shown in the figure.

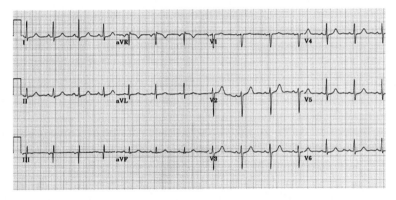

Figure 13.5   Normal 12-channel ECG. (Image courtesy of Dean Jenkins, ECG Library.)[1]

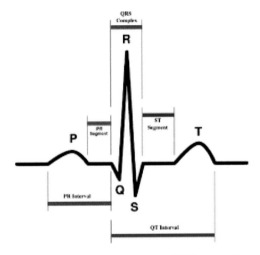

Figure 13.6   The P-Q-R-S-T complex. Basic ECG waveforms, intervals, and segments. (Creative Commons Attribution-ShareAlike, 4.0 license)[2]

Electrocardiography is the technique to produce an electrocardiogram (ECG), a recording of the heart's electrical activity. It is an electrogram of the heart, which is a graph of voltage versus time of the electrical activity of the heart using electrodes placed on the skin. These electrodes detect the small electrical changes that are a consequence of cardiac muscle depolarization followed by repolarization during each cardiac cycle, a heartbeat. Changes in the normal ECG pattern occur in numerous cardiac abnormalities, including cardiac rhythm disturbances, such as ventricular tachycardia (a type of abnormal heart rhythm, or arrhythmia); inadequate coronary artery blood flow (such as myocardial ischemia and myocardial infarction); and electrolyte disturbances, such as hypokalemia (low level of potassium [K⁺] in the blood) and hyperkalemia (elevated level of potassium [K⁺] in the blood).

Traditionally, ECG usually means a 12-lead ECG taken while lying down, as discussed later. However, other devices can record the electrical activity of the heart, such as a Holter monitor (a type of portable electrocardiography device), but also some models of smartwatches/smartphones are capable of recording an ECG.

In a conventional 12-lead ECG, 10 electrodes are placed on the patient's limbs and on the surface of the chest. The overall magnitude of the heart's electrical potential is then measured from twelve different angles (leads) and is recorded over a period (usually 10 seconds). In this way, the overall magnitude and direction of the heart's electrical depolarization are captured at each moment throughout the cardiac cycle.

There are three main components to an ECG: the P wave, which represents the depolarization of the atria; the QRS-complex, which represents the depolarization of the ventricles; and the T wave, which represents the repolarization of the ventricles.[3]

13.1.2   Blood Pressure Measurements

Blood pressure is one of the parameters included in what is called the vital signs (Figure 13.7). There are four parameters included in the basic set of vital signs: blood pressure, temperature, pulse (heart rate), and breathing rate.

The basic list of vital signs is mission-critical in all lifesaving health situations. This enables nurses and doctors to know the next step in a lifesaving procedure. As you can see in the longer list in Figure 13.7, there are

Vital Sign	Physiology	Influencing Factor
Temperature	Controlled by hypothalamus	Age, infection, medication
Pulse	Reflects circulation and volume strength of contractility	Intravascular volume, contractility, oxygen demand
Blood pressure	Regulated by vasomotor center in the medula	Intravascular volume, vascular tone, contractility
Respiratory rate	Controlled by the respiratory centers in the medula and pons	Hypercapnia, hypoxemia, acidosis
SpO₂	Reflects the peripheral saturation of hemoglobin by O₂	Cardiac output; hemoglobin level of fraction of inspired O₂
Pain	Detected by peripheral nerve fibers: interpreted by thalamus and cerebral cortex	Patient's perception
Level of consciousnes	Controlled by reticular activating system in the brain stem	Cerebral perfusion
Urine output	Produced by kidneys	Cardiac output; hemoglobin level of fraction of inspired O₂

Figure 13.7   Vital signs. (Own design, with data mainly from en.wikipedia.org)

additional parameters that healthcare professionals need or would like to know, if it is possible, in the actual situation.[4]

Blood tests: Blood tests are often used in healthcare to determine physiological and biochemical states, such as disease, mineral content, pharmaceutical drug effectiveness, and organ function. Typical clinical blood panels include a basic metabolic panel or a complete blood count. Blood tests are also used in drug tests to detect drug abuse.

The number of tests that are available today is more than 300 different tests. They differ in sensitivity and specificity, but hardly any doctor's visit happens without a relatively long list of blood tests being executed.

Blood tests are probably the most common diagnostic test method today.[5]

13.1.3   Pacemaker

The primary purpose of a pacemaker (Figure 13.8) is to maintain an adequate heart rate, either because the heart's natural pacemaker is not fast enough or because there is a block in the heart's electrical conduction system. Modern pacemakers are externally programmable and allow a cardiologist to select the optimum pacing modes for individual patients. Modern devices are demand pacemakers, in which the stimulation of the heart is based on the dynamic demand of the circulatory system. A major step forward in pacemaker function has been to attempt to mimic nature by utilizing various inputs to produce a rate-responsive pacemaker using parameters such as the QT interval pO_2–pCO_2 (dissolved oxygen or carbon dioxide levels) in the arterial-venous system, physical activity as determined by an accelerometer, body temperature ATP levels, and adrenaline. Instead

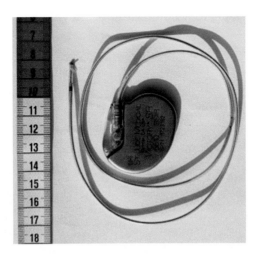

Figure 13.8   Pacemaker. (en.wikipedia.org)

of producing a static, predetermined heart rate, or intermittent control, such a pacemaker, a dynamic pacemaker, could compensate for both actual respiratory loading and potentially anticipated respiratory loading. The first dynamic pacemaker was invented by Anthony Rickards of the National Heart Hospital, London, UK, in 1982.[6]

Figure 13.9 shows posteroanterior and lateral chest radiographs of a pacemaker with normally located leads in the right atrium (white arrow) and right ventricle (black arrowhead), respectively.

The first static pacemaker was developed by the Swedish engineer Rune Elmqvist in 1958 and implanted in a patient in 1960.[7]

13.1.4   Heart Starter/Defibrillators

Defibrillators are devices that send an electric pulse or shock to the heart to restore a normal heartbeat. They are used to prevent or correct an arrhythmia, an uneven heartbeat that is too slow or too fast. If the heart suddenly stops, defibrillators can also help it beat again.

Today, you can get a combination of a pacemaker and a defibrillator implanted in case your heart problems are more of a chronic nature.

Today, heart starters are available in most official places where people meet. The units today are extremely simple to use, and non-medically trained people can operate them.[8]

13.1.5   Mobile ECG

The drawback with the conventional ECG approach is that it only gives a rather short observation time of the ECG. It is normally a but limited measurement during maybe 10–20-seconds, and many different heart events, of course, happens outside this time frame. New developments in ECG measurements, like mobile ECG (Figure 13.10), can register an ECG for a person or patient while in action instead of lying on a couch for a minute

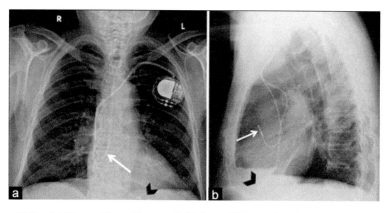

Figure 13.9   (a) Frontal lung X-ray and (b) lateral X-ray of an implanted pacemaker.
(en.wikipedia.org)

or so. The mobile version can also be used to measure long-term ECGs. Unfortunately, long-term ECGs also put a tough demand on the doctor doing the analysis. Developments are ongoing for automatic analysis using artificial intelligence (AI) in order to reduce the challenges for doctors to read and analyze long-term ECGs. This will enable more practical long-term ECG use.

Many new applications for healthcare are available or will become available on the smartphones available today (Figure 13.11).

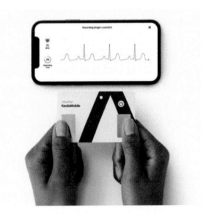

Figure 13.10   Mobile ECG with a smartphone and channel ECG. (www.dovepress. com; Creative Commons Attribution-NonCommercial [unported, v3.0] License)[9]

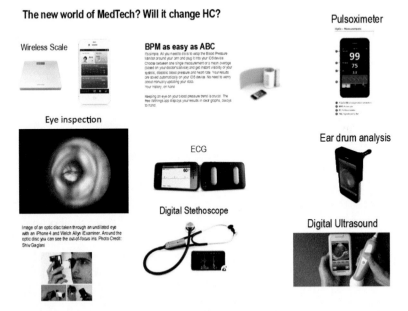

Figure 13.11   A growing number of applications will be introduced to our smartphones. (*Note:* Some of these apparatus and technologies have not been validated, to my knowledge.) (www.bcbi.nlm.nih.gov.pmc)[10]

13.1.6   Atrial Fibrillation Detection

Atrial fibrillation (AF) is not considered to be a serious health issue if you are otherwise in good health. If you have other health problems, like diabetes, high blood pressure, or other diseases of the heart, atrial fibrillation can be dangerous. Either way, this condition needs to be properly diagnosed and managed by a doctor.

A 12-lead ECG recording is the gold standard to confirm an AF diagnosis. This method is well suited for patients with continuous and rather stable AF. For patients with only apparent AF, several new mobile techniques are more effective.

Figure 13.11 shows some of the many new techniques adapted to a smartphone. These techniques are becoming more and more competent, and more new techniques are being added. Soon, this will allow the distribution of a lot of new methods to smaller clinics and into our homes, enabling self-diagnostics remotely, which can then be read by your doctor.[11]

13.1.7   Clinical Chemical Analytical Equipment

Clinical chemistry is used to analyze samples from patients to gather information about their health and tailor a treatment protocol for them. Clinical chemistry is used in medical labs, research labs, pharmaceutical companies, and academic labs. Some of the many clinical chemistry instruments used to gather information for health analysis are microscopes; blood analyzers, including cell counters; electrolyte, glucose, and oxygen analyzers; equipment for urinalysis; various immunoassays; and gel electrophoresis equipment for analyzing DNA. Clinical chemistry instruments allow scientists to determine properties in blood, urine, stool, tissues, and even DNA that can help them pinpoint the patient's problem and how to best treat it.[12]

13.1.8   Biopsy Tools

Tissue or cell samples can be taken from almost any part of the body. How samples are taken depends on where the tumor is and what type of cancer is suspected. For instance, the methods used for skin biopsies are very different from those used for brain biopsies.

Some types of biopsies remove an entire organ. These are only done by surgeons. Other types of biopsies remove tumor samples through a thin needle or through an endoscope (a flexible lighted tube that's put into the body). These biopsies are often done by surgeons but can also be done by other doctors.[13]

Fine needle biopsy (sometimes called fine needle aspiration, FNA): FNA uses a very thin, hollow needle attached to a syringe to take out a small amount of fluid and very small pieces of tissue from the tumor. The doctor can aim the needle while feeling the tumor, if it's near the surface of the body. If the tumor is deeper inside the body and can't be felt, the needle can be guided while being watched on an imaging test, such as an ultrasound or CT scan.[14]

Core needle biopsy (also called core biopsy): Needles used in a core biopsy are slightly larger than those used in FNA. They remove a small cylinder of tissue (about 1/16 inch or approximately 0.16 mm in diameter and 1.27 mm long). The core needle biopsy is done with local anesthesia (drugs are used to make the area insensitive) in the doctor's office or clinic. Like FNA, a core biopsy can sample tumors that the doctor can feel as well as smaller ones that must be seen using imaging tests.[14]

13.1.9   Pathological Analytical Tools

A pathology laboratory is a laboratory where tests are carried out on clinical specimens to obtain information about the health of a patient to aid in the diagnosis, treatment, and prevention of disease.

The Pathologist is a new tool designed to transform large sets of gene expression data into quantitative descriptors of pathway-level behavior. The tool aims to provide a robust alternative to the search for single-gene-to-phenotype associations by accounting for the complexity of molecular interactions.

Recent biomedical research has made great strides in unveiling the complexity of human disease. Technological breakthroughs and innovative methodologies now allow a much more detailed account of molecular behavior. Frequently, however, such studies yield a plethora of data, with results too complex for traditional analyses designed to identify single genes associated with diseases.[15, 16]

Reference List, Chapter 13

1 Image Courtesy Dean Jenkins, ECG Library. Normal 12 channel ECG
2 www.wikilectures.eu/w/Electrocardiogram
3 www.sciencedirect.com/science/article/pii/S0213911121002466
4 Own Design, data from https://en.wikipedia.org/wiki/Vital_signs
5 www.nhs.uk/conditions/blood-tests/
6 https://en.wikipedia.org/wiki/Artificial_cardiac_pacemaker
7 https://en.wikipedia.org/wiki/Artificial_cardiac_pacemaker
8 https://en.wikipedia.org/wiki/Defibrillation
9 www.dovepress.com/smartphone-electrocardiogram-monitoring-current-perspectives-peer-reviewed-fulltext-article-AHCT
10 www.ncbi.nlm.nih.gov/pmc/articles/PMC4029126/
11 www.nhs.uk/conditions/atrial-fibrillation/diagnosis/
12 www.labcompare.com/Clinical-Diagnostics/5127-Clinical-Chemistry-Instruments/
13 www.researchgate.net/figure/Instruments-used-in-skin-biopsy-procedures_fig1_221918815
14 www.nhs.uk/conditions/biopsy/what-happens/
15 www.med.upenn.edu/dac/pathology-analytics.html
16 www.sciencedirect.com/science/article/abs/pii/0169260794900930

14

MEDICINE AND MEDICAL TECHNOLOGY BUSINESSES

Let's have a look at the business and business models within healthcare technologies. The business part is extremely important for new developments within medicine and MedTech in order to reach patients for improved care and to reach the general public for preventive purposes. The continuous exchange of technology and methods is at a reasonable pace following the new applications being launched.

At the beginning of my hospital physicist experience at the Linköping University Hospital, we developed new technical ideas and tools internally within the technical/physics team (this was from 1972 onward), and then we went to the clinicians and asked if they could use what we had created.

My experience is that this old-fashioned way has changed gradually year by year. Today, most of the questions originate from clinical problems and requests. With this focus, from the start, it is already obvious what type of expertise will be needed for a specific project. Certainly, as a project progresses, there are always new developments that will need additional expertise, but the basic knowledge is already there when the project goals are defined.

Many of the research teams of today are built from the beginning with most of the needed competencies (Figure 14.1). Good examples of building diversified and strong competency teams are the European research framework programs under the European Union, Horizon 2020, and the latest one, Horizon Europe, introduced in January 2021.

Today, the key to progress and success is through collaboration. For many of us who have participated in these research programs, we have seen progress and been able to witness the collaborative spirit and stimulation of these EU initiatives. I am also very convinced that by the way that these research frameworks are organized, they have led to important research results and will continue to do so.

Another important parameter for the continued success of these research frameworks is the fact that both small and medium companies (SMEs), together with large companies, can participate in the EU framework research funding programs. The result has been that research has had a clear goal not only to enable good research but to enable the healthcare research to reach the commercial and product phase and, ultimately, the hospitals and the patients.

DOI: 10.1201/9781003393320-17

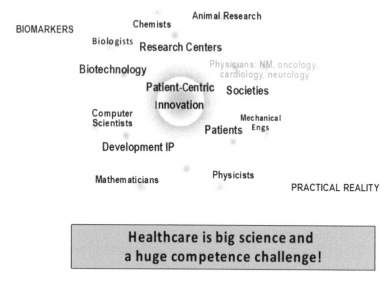

Many different competencies are needed in modern healthcare developments

BIOMARKERS

Chemists

Animal Research

Biologists   Research Centers

Biotechnology

Physicians: NM, oncology,
cardiology, neurology

Patient-Centric   Societies

Innovation

Computer
Scientists   Mechanical
                             Engs
                    Patients

Development IP

Mathematicians   Physicists

                              PRACTICAL REALITY

Healthcare is big science and
a huge competence challenge!

Figure 14.1 Example of the needed competencies in modern medicine and MedTech development. (Courtesy of Bengt Långström; collaboration between Bengt Långström and Bengt Nielsen.)[1]

The fact that small and medium companies, together with large companies, can participate has brought a more realistic view of the very long lead times in MedTech. It has also brought muscles in the form of money to the cost side of the equation. We must not forget the importance these collaborations have meant for companies, and getting insight into the future research in technical as well as diagnostic and treatment ideas is mission-critical for all parties. Developments need to be focused on the needs of the healthcare side.

This type of development, with several parties collaborating, is sometimes called triple helix collaborations, aiming for collaboration among academia (universities), government, and industries.

During the research and development process, there are mainly three stakeholders that need to get their arms around their different priorities. The government/society's role is, at this stage, more in the background.

The road from the point of having a device with technical ability is very long for all biomedical engineering tools under development. It can still take another 15–20 years. For Sweden, the equivalent mean time to market is 17 years on average.

There are several reasons why it takes such a long time to develop, market, and launch MedTech products.

The initial thing to realize is that the regulatory landscape is tough, as the technology is developed for patients. Therefore the regulations must be very strict.

The development normally starts with an idea for a specific task. Rather quickly, you may even have a prototype. Then it is very common in the MedTech field that overly optimistic hype is built. Challenges normally come when raising funding. When the regulatory and validation process starts, most teams and companies realize that the time it takes to manage the process normally takes much more time than planned, and this can easily become twice or three times what is in the original plan.

These are a few of the reasons why the development time and, thereby, costs are a challenge within MedTech.

14.1   Drug Discovery and Development

Drug discovery is challenging, as it has some very demanding quality control steps to follow. The demand for safety is very strict, and hence, this is driving the cost side upward.

> *Discovery phase:* This can take many years of research, and 2–10 years is very common. This phase starts with the screening of 5,000 to 10,000 samples.
>
> *Preclinical testing:* Laboratory and animal testing. Before going into animal testing, the number of samples has been screened down to a number of approximately 250.
>
> *Phase I:* 20–80 healthy volunteers; used to determine safety and dosage.
>
> *Phase II:* 100–300 patient volunteers; used to look for efficacy and side effects. Before starting the clinical test, the number of candidates has been brought down to approximately five sample compound candidates.
>
> *Phase III:* 1,000–5,000 patient volunteers; used to monitor adverse reactions to long-term use.
>
> *FDA review approval:* Additional postmarketing testing.[2]

The time frame for development is very similar to developments within biomedical engineering. The main difference is the cost side of the developments. Drug developments normally cost 10–15 times more than biomedical engineering projects. The main reason for this difference has been the regulatory process that has been applied within drug development. Today, the regulatory process for MedTech is more similar to the pharmaceutical one, and hence, the differences are less pronounced.

Personal Anecdote

During my time at GE HealthCare when I was responsible for our external research projects where we collaborated with leading universities and hospitals, primarily in Europe, I organized yearly research meetings between our key partners and our top management at the GE HealthCare headquarters in London. At one of these meetings, we had a representative from Pfizer pharmaceuticals. He told us that if we, GE HealthCare, could help Pfizer with methods and technologies in order to stop drug development projects at an earlier step than when they reach phase 3, we would be highly credited. It is rare that someone in the commercial side of things wants help to halt projects.

The reason is that when a potential drug candidate reaches phase 3, the cost of the development reaches many millions of dollars. Pfizer needed methods and processes in order to kill the project that was less viable in favor of the one that was highly viable. The fact that the pharmaceutical industry continued too long with drug candidates that would fail in the end gave rise to big losses, preventing new and more viable investments.

14.2   Drivers in Today's Medicine and Technologies

Every period has its own drivers for new developments (Figure 14.2). In the 21st century, we are seeing great progress through information technology developments, like supercomputing and internet mobile applications, and medical imaging technology. Additionally, we are seeing great steps being taken within molecular medicine and within biology. Technology developments also make it possible to start using genomics in clinical practice, not only for research applications. All these new areas of will enable an even faster development phase.

The number of artificial intelligence (AI) projects and applications in all categories of development is visible everywhere today. For many applications, there are clear advantages. Some applications, though, are more questionable and need a deeper analysis of what the benefits are or will become.

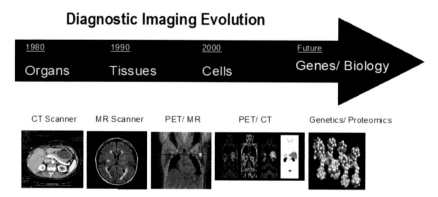

Figure 14.2   The diagnostic imaging evolution. (Courtesy of Bengt Långström; collaboration between Bengt Långström and Bengt Nielsen.)[3]

The new step in the imaging evolution is how we will start moving forward in exploring biology with expanding genomics and proteomics tools.

Another important step in imaging is that the different imaging techniques are becoming gradually more functional and not only delivering morphological images of an organ/tissue.

Moreover, each modality is also becoming more quantitative in order for the radiologist/clinician to give answers based on quantitative data and not only by qualitative answers.

The trend to combine modalities in order to increase specificity is clearly seen when a PET is combined with a CT. The CT is great for localizing an organ or tissue, while the PET is able to tell us what type of tissue or tumor we see in the image. This clearly improves the specificity.

When we combine different modalities with AI, we will be able to deliver much more robust diagnostic information and, at the same time, more quickly. More on AI is available in Chapter 21.

Reference List, Chapter 14

1 Collaboration between Bengt Långström and Bengt Nielsen, Example of Needed Competences in Modern Medicine and MedTech Development
2 www.sciencedirect.com/journal/drug-discovery-today/articles-in-press
3 Collaboration between Bengt Långström and Bengt Nielsen, The Diagnostic Imaging Evolution

15

MEDICAL BIOMARKERS, CRITICAL TOOLS TODAY AND TOMORROW

15.1 Stratify to Justify

I can't remember when I heard this expression the first time. It does not origin from me, but I like the concept. Most likely, the expression was given to me by Prof. Harry Holthöfer, Helsinki, Finland.

Today, we can diagnose many different diseases, and the techniques we have provide both sensitivity and specificity. The challenge we face continuously is that we cannot put every person on our planet through all the possible tests and diagnostic procedures we can offer today and in the future. We will need to prioritize those individuals that most likely need to be tested. We will need to define and work according to some strategy, to avoid trying to end up in a mission impossible situation or like "boiling the ocean".

What we can possibly offer today and in the future are simplified tests or existing data from a person's medical history in order to identify persons at risk for a certain disease.

By working along these lines, the number of persons with a risk for a certain diagnosis becomes a bit more manageable to execute in the practical situation. Moreover, it is these persons whom we want to offer care first.

In Figure 20.1, the example chosen is Alzheimer's disease. In this case, a PET exam could potentially answer the questions for clinical evidence of either mild cognitive impairment (MCI) or Alzheimer's disease (AD).

A PET exam is a rather exclusive investigation in the sense that it cannot be done at all hospitals. Ongoing research is moving forward fast, and today, it is becoming possible to diagnose AD through a rather simple blood test. With a simple blood test, AD diagnosis becomes much more realistic to diagnose in a rather large population without having to put all the potential candidates into a PET camera.

Let's hope that the blood test for AD will become available within a couple of years. Right now, the method is looking very promising. Several research groups around the world are working on this important task.

15.2 Definition

In medicine, a biomarker is a measurable indicator of a malfunction or the presence of some disease state. More generally, a biomarker is anything that can be used as an indicator of a particular disease state or some

DOI: 10.1201/9781003393320-18

other physiological state of an organism. According to the WHO, the indicator may be chemical, physical, or biological in nature. The measurement may be functional, physiological, biochemical, cellular, or molecular. The term *biomarker* actually stands for "biological marker." So as the word itself suggests, a biomarker is a measurable marker or sign that tells a medical professional what is taking place inside a patient's body. A biomarker can be a sign, relatively easy to observe, such as a patient's blood pressure level, or it can also be a marker/indicator that requires more complex testing to detect, for example, the presence of a certain protein in a patient's blood.

A biomarker can also be a substance that is introduced into an organism as a means to examine organ function or other aspects of health. For example, rubidium chloride (RbCl) is used in isotopic labeling to evaluate the perfusion of the heart muscle. It can also be a substance whose detection indicates a particular disease state; for example, the presence of an antibody may indicate an infection.

More specifically, a biomarker can indicate a change in the expression or state of a protein that correlates with the risk or progression of a disease. It could also correspond with the susceptibility of the disease to a given treatment.

Biomarkers can be characteristic biological properties or molecules that can be detected and measured in parts of the body, like in the blood or specific tissue. Biomarkers may indicate either normal or diseased processes in the body and can be specific cells, molecules, genes, gene products, enzymes, or hormones.

Complex organ functions or general characteristic changes in biological structures can also serve as biomarkers.

Although the term *biomarker* is relatively new, biomarkers have been used in preclinical research and clinical diagnosis for a considerable time. For example, body temperature is a well-known biomarker for fever. Blood pressure is used to determine the risk of stroke. It is also widely known that cholesterol values are a biomarker and risk indicator for coronary and vascular diseases and that C-reactive protein (CRP) is a marker for inflammation.

Biomarkers are very useful in several ways, including measuring the progress of diseases, evaluating the most effective therapeutic regimes for a particular cancer type, and establishing long-term susceptibility to cancer or its recurrence.

The parameter can be chemical, physical, or biological.

In molecular terms, *biomarker* is "the subset of markers" that might be discovered using genomics, proteomics, or imaging technologies. Biomarkers play major roles in medicinal biology. Biomarkers help in early diagnosis, disease prevention, drug target identification, drug response, and more.

We will also look at specific biomarkers for different diseases in cardiovascular events.

For drug development industries, biomarkers are mission-critical in order to indicate and quantify the efficacy of drug candidates as well as be able to verify that a drug has reached the intended target.

Several biomarkers have been identified for many diseases, such as serum LDL for cholesterol, blood pressure, and the P53 gene.

MMPs (matrix metalloproteinases), like MMP-9, are found to be important in relation to the pathology of cancers and tumor markers for cancer, including metastasis and angiogenesis.

MMPs are also thought to play a major role in cell behavior, such as cell migration, adhesion/dispersion, differentiation, angiogenesis, apoptosis (cell death), and host defense.[1]

The ultimate goals for research focused on complex human diseases are to either prevent or cure the diseases. These are very ambitious goals that will be greatly facilitated by the identification of new biomarkers that can serve as novel diagnostic or prognostic indicators of disease course, that can be used as surrogate disease markers to track the efficacy of novel treatment strategies, or that may provide new targets for the treatment of the diseases.

15.3   Different Categories of Biomarkers

Different biomarkers are used for different purposes. The US Food and Drug Administration (FDA) and the National Institutes of Health (NIH) in the United States have jointly published a glossary defining each biomarker type.

15.3.1   *Diagnostic Biomarkers*

Just like the results of a mechanic's diagnostic tests, a diagnostic biomarker indicates the presence of a specific medical condition or disease in a patient's body. It is a valuable tool that enables doctors to make more precise diagnoses. As mentioned earlier, no reliable diagnostic biomarker has been found to work as an early detector for ovarian cancer.

15.3.2   *Monitoring Biomarkers*

A monitoring biomarker is a biomarker that is assessed repeatedly over time to keep track of how a disease is progressing, much like continually checking the oil level of a leaky car. Since biomarkers can be measured, a doctor can monitor them over the course of weeks, months, and years to see if a patient's condition is improving, staying the same, or worsening.

In addition to helping a doctor simply keep watch on the progression of a medical condition, a monitoring biomarker can also tell a doctor how the disease is responding to treatment. This characteristic is particularly valuable because it shows doctors what is working or not working. This type of information, in turn, helps doctors provide their patients with more effective therapies.

Cancer antigen 125 (CA-125) is a biomarker for ovarian cancer. It is primarily considered a monitoring biomarker for ovarian cancer that doctors use to keep watch on how well an ovarian cancer treatment is working for a patient. Since CA-125 is released into the bloodstream, levels are measured via a blood test.

15.3.3   Predictive Biomarkers

Another tool used to tailor a patient's care plan is the predictive biomarker. This biomarker type can be used by doctors to identify which individuals will respond best to treatment.

Remember the oil-leaky car? Perhaps the auto mechanic is aware of a specific design quirk that is known to cause leaks in this car model.

That knowledge will give the mechanic useful insight into how best to fix the leak. In much the same way, a predictive biomarker, such as a gene mutation, can provide a doctor with crucial information as to whether a treatment is more or less likely to work for a particular patient.

When a patient has been diagnosed with ovarian cancer, a doctor may test for predictive biomarkers, such as BRCA and other cancer-causing gene mutations. Detected through blood or saliva tests, these mutations can signal to a doctor what therapies may work best for that patient.

15.3.4   Susceptibility/Risk Biomarkers

Gene mutations can also function as susceptibility/risk biomarkers. These biomarkers can point to the probability of a disease or medical condition developing well before it is present in the body, much like how a manufacturing glitch in a car model can serve as a warning sign that the engine may fail in the future. In the case of BRCA gene mutations, they can alert the doctor to the risk of ovarian or other types of cancers developing. And depending on the risk level for ovarian cancer specifically, the doctor may recommend preventive measures, such as removing a patient's ovaries and/or fallopian tubes.

15.3.5   Prognostic Biomarkers

Another biomarker category that helps provide a doctor with a more well-defined picture of a patient's future is the prognostic biomarker. A doctor may use this type of biomarker after the diagnosis of a disease to determine how the patient's condition may progress without factoring in therapy. A prognostic biomarker gives clues as to the likelihood of a patient experiencing a future recurrence or the development of a new medical condition.

In the field of ovarian cancer research, there are two proteins that show promise as prognostic biomarkers, though research in this area is ongoing. These proteins, which can be found in both healthy and cancerous cells, are called progesterone receptors (PR) and estrogen receptors (ER). The presence of progesterone receptors and/or estrogen receptors in cancerous cells has been linked to higher survival rates for patients living with certain types of ovarian cancer.

15.3.6   Typical Biomarkers That Are Used Today

- Alanine transaminase (ALT)
- Body fat percentage
- Body mass index
- Body temperature
- Blood pressure
- Blood sugar level
- Complete blood count
- Creatinine
- C-reactive protein/inflammation
- Heart rate
- Hematocrit (HCT)
- Hemoglobin (Hgb)
- Mean corpuscular volume (MCV)
- Red blood cell count (RBC)
- Thyroid-stimulating hormone (TSH)
- Triglyceride
- Waist circumference
- Waist-to-hip ratio (WHR)

15.3.7   Biomarkers in Cancer

Biomarkers have contributed to lifesaving breakthroughs in cancer detection and treatments. They are a critical tool in medical research, as they help scientists get a better understanding of what biological factors may cause different cancers, which investigational drugs are most effective in combatting the disease, and how specific therapies should be targeted once approved.

When scientists study cancer biomarkers, they are typically observing signs on a molecular level. These markers, which may include proteins and genes, are so tiny that they cannot be seen with the naked eye. Cancer biomarkers may exist in the tumor cells themselves as well as in other cells of the body that are reacting to cancer.

15.3.8   Biomarkers in Cardiovascular Events

There are several clinical biomarkers that are associated with cardiovascular diseases or events:

- *Cardiac troponin* is a protein, and it is by far the most commonly used biomarker and has very high sensitivity. In three to four hours after myocardial infarction, it is released into the blood circulation system and remains detectable for up to 10 days.

- *Myoglobin* is a common biomarker for myocardial infarction. Myoglobin is released into the circulation system within 30 minutes of an injury.
- *Creatine kinase*—also known as creatine phosphokinase or CPK—is a muscle enzyme that exists as iso-enzymes (enzymes that differ in amino acid sequence but catalyze the same chemical reactions). Iso-enzymes usually have different kinetic parameters (different KM values or are regulated differently).

15.3.9   Neurological Biomarkers

Neurological biomarkers are detectable substances primarily found in the cerebrospinal fluid (CSF) when there has been some damage to the brain. These biomarkers help in the early diagnosis of neurological disorders, drug development, and personalized medicine development.

The growing research and discovery in the field of neurology have enabled the introduction of novel methods for the detection and better treatment of neurological disorders, such as Alzheimer's disease, schizophrenia, and Parkinson's disease.

There are primarily four groups of biomarkers within neurology applications.

15.3.10   Imaging Biomarkers

MRI and PET imaging are the primary techniques here. For Parkinson's disease, SPECT imaging with DatScan can help in diagnosing Parkinson's disease, but a clinical exam by a neurologist can make the diagnosis with the same accuracy.

Although imaging biomarkers play a key role in the central nervous system, they should be used in conjunction with other biomarkers, such as blood-based, CSF-based, genetic, and electrophysiological biomarkers. This is in order to increase the specificity of the biomarker.

15.3.11   Metabolomics Biomarkers

Definition: *Metabolomics* is defined as the systematic study of all chemical processes concerning metabolites, providing characteristic chemical fingerprints that specific cellular processes yield, by means of the study of their small-molecule metabolite profiles.

Metabolomics is an analytical profiling technique for measuring and comparing large numbers of metabolites present in biological samples.

Combining high-throughput analytical chemistry and multivariate data analysis, metabolomics offers a window into metabolic mechanisms. Because they intimately utilize and often rewire host metabolism, viruses are an excellent choice to study by metabolomics techniques.[2]

15.3.12   Proteomics Biomarkers

Proteomic biomarkers are often referred to as those biomarkers discovered using technologies capable of analyzing many proteins simultaneously, such as protein microarray and mass spectrometry (MS).

15.3.13   Genomics Biomarkers

Definition: A measurable DNA and/or RNA characteristic that is an indicator of normal biologic processes, pathogenic processes, and/or response to therapeutic or other interventions.

Technology for high-throughput scanning of the human genome and its encoded proteins has rapidly developed to allow systematic analyses of human disease. The application of these technologies is becoming an increasingly effective approach for identifying the biological basis of genetically complex neurological diseases.

The arsenal of biomarkers in neurology is likely to keep growing as our ability to accurately measure multiple biological variables and our knowledge about the pathophysiology of neurological diseases increase.[3]

Why do we need and want to understand how our genes work and how our proteins build our bodies?

All human individuals' sets of DNA and proteins are unique. We will eventually be able to give all patients a treatment that is adapted to their own specific genetic conditions.

Today, the sequencing of a person's complete genome takes about 1–2 days. It is expected that this time will become shorter and shorter. The increased speed enables our healthcare system to use genetic data for improved diagnosis and therapeutics. The most-used applications today are within cancer diagnosis, giving potential for individual treatment.

In Sweden, the project Genomic Medicine Sweden was introduced a few years ago. This initiative/project will spread the knowledge and the methodology to the whole country. This is the start of precision medicine in Sweden. The first applications are cancer and unusual hereditary diseases:

Phase 1: Discovery research
Phase 2: Testing and adaption for diagnosis
Phase 3: Diagnostic validation and implementation
Phase 4: Clinical diagnostics

The leadership for the research parts of the project belongs to SciLifeLab Clinical Genomics, an organization of the Royal Technical University; the seven healthcare regions in the country; and the seven universities that belong to the seven regions (www.nature.com/articles/s41591-022-01963-4).

In Sweden, the key to the successful implementation of precision medicine in healthcare has been the bottom-up approach, where academia and healthcare have joined forces to build a national infrastructure.

Forty-two authors from the Clinical Genomics platform at Califia (National/International Infrastructure in Lund, specialized in detectors) and Genomic Medicine Sweden (GMS) summarized the work in *Nature Medicine*.

Together, Clinical Genomics and GMS have established an innovative framework for continuously developing, adapting, and implementing precision medicine in healthcare, for all patients. At the seven locations in Sweden with a faculty of medicine and regional healthcare providers with university hospital care, both Clinical Genomics and GMS have established nodes to facilitate the development and optimization of new technologies and methods and their introduction into healthcare throughout the country.[4]

15.4   Footnote

Genotyping is the process of determining differences in the genetic makeup (genotype) of an individual by examining the individual's DNA using modern sequencing techniques.

The genotype–phenotype distinction is drawn in genetics. Genotype is an organism's full hereditary information. Phenotype is an organism's actual observed properties, such as morphology, development, or behavior. This distinction is fundamental in the study of the inheritance of traits and their evolution.[5]

Reference List, Chapter 15

1 https://en.wikipedia.org/wiki/Matrix_metalloproteinase
2 https://pubmed.ncbi.nlm.nih.gov/28433052/ Marianne Manchester, Anisha Anand, in Advances in Virus Research, 2017
3 www.science.org/content/article/biomarkers-brain-putting-biomarkers-together-better-understanding-nervous-system
4 https://genomicmedicine.se in Swedish & English
5 https://monogrambio.labcorp.com/resources/genotyping-vs-phenotyping

Part 4

THE FUTURE

16

OUR HEALTHCARE SYSTEM

16.1 Our Healthcare Foundation Is Changing

- Discoveries in bioscience open new possibilities:
  - Human genomics is known
  - Proteomics: Human Protein Atlas is ready
  - Biomarkers and biosensors
- More than 50% of all drugs have no effect on the prescribed disease* or effects on the patient

Responders and non-responders need to be identified.

- The Digital Revolution is ongoing
- The patient will own his own diagnosis and treatment
- Lack of healthcare professionals is becoming a limiting factor all over the world
- Chronic diseases are ticking bombs: Lifestyle changes are needed. Most cardiovascular diseases could be dramatically reduced by changes in our lifestyle
- Approximately 80% of coronary heart disease, up to 90% of type 2 diabetes, and more than 50% of all cancers could be prevented through lifestyle changes, such as proper diet and exercise[1, 2]

Note: The previously mentioned data are a bit old, and I have been working on getting newer data. I have not managed to find any newer data unfortunately.

Financing modern healthcare has become a huge challenge and a continuous discussion around the world. Should healthcare be a responsibility of the individual or should it be granted by the governments and paid for via taxes like in Scandinavia or should it be some type of combination?

Or maybe we all need to incorporate health insurance in our private budget in order to guarantee our routine healthcare?

Healthcare demands and needs will always be higher than what any healthcare system has the capacity for or will be able to offer. This is the same all over the world, independent of how different countries around the world have solved or built their health service.

DOI: 10.1201/9781003393320-20

We will be able to diagnose and treat more and more diseases, and our healthcare systems around the world will be even more stretched and challenged on the cost side. In order to keep healthcare at an affordable level for people, we will probably have to make some rather tough priorities in the future. Maybe one way is that we will have to comply with lifestyle changes in case of very expensive treatments.

The rapid change and need for new technology have further added both the money and training needs of personnel as we move forward. The technical lifetime of new diagnostic and therapeutic equipment is rather short, and consequently, this will lead to large investment demands for today's hospitals and clinics in the rich world. For the developing world, the challenges ahead of them are even more demanding, as they are in a different situation, building their healthcare systems from scratch, in many countries.

The principle for any healthcare system must be that the patients with the most medical needs should be prioritized. The challenge everywhere is in making this prioritizing process happen in practice. Many different methodologies have been tried. In the past, these were mainly based on telephone service, using nurses and doctors to make the challenging calls of prioritization and seeing to it that everyone is waiting in the right lane for their needs. The healthcare service NHS in the UK, for instance, used this method during the 1990s with mixed success.

Remember that everyone living in the world does not have access to the level of healthcare we are talking about. When and how the countries that are behind will be able to catch up is not easy to predict.

In Sweden, we are known to have a world-class healthcare service, while we are often struggling with how to organize primary care so that not all patients end up in a very long queue for specialist care. Everybody is demanding more resources—primary care as well as specialist care. Should primary care have more specialists or should specialist care be expanded? How do we offer the same high-level care all over a country and at the same time guarantee that every patient is diagnosed and treated within reasonable time limits and without unnecessary waiting time?

Probably many countries are thinking very much along the same lines.

In the future, we hope to have new and improved digital tools to manage and ease the critical bottleneck of selecting and prioritizing patients with acute and real healthcare needs. Later, some modern ideas for digital care will be discussed.

16.2   Care Models Combining Virtual and In-Person Services

The Covid-19 pandemic (2019–2022) and the need for physical distancing were responsible for a major acceleration of virtual care over the last two years. According to a market report (July 2021, McKinsey & Company), the market could reach US$250 billion.

Virtual care and telehealth are here to stay; and do not incorporate in-person care, however. Instead, we can expect to see more of a hybrid solution, as care providers seek to offer patients the best of both worlds.

Patients can expect to be encouraged to do more initial and simple consultations via digital calls, wherein they describe issues to a doctor or nurse, who can then assess need and schedule a visit or tests accordingly. Those with common conditions, such as minor infections or flu, can go over symptoms and be issued a prescription.

Refills of prescriptions can mostly be done by simply sending an email via a patient portal.

For times when a doctor needs to conduct a physical examination or when tests need to be performed, in-person care will remain as usual. This hybridization will save time for patients and care professionals alike, making the processes—from arranging appointments to doing follow-ups—more efficient and convenient.

The demand for healthcare will always be above the capabilities of a given society, and the critical issue is to be able to prioritize access to the needed and relevant healthcare service for the people with the highest needs.

This is probably one of the biggest challenges, being able to make this selection correctly and efficiently.

16.3   What Can Artificial Intelligence Do within Healthcare?

When it comes to AI in healthcare, it's safe to say technology cannot replace a human doctor. Doctors still offer the best judgment and experience in treating members of the public.

With respect to population health, which has become even more important since the pandemic, AI is needed more than ever to provide help and support for the diagnosis and treatment statistics and other information to specialists and public health researchers.

Population health management software typically integrates patient data across healthcare IT systems for analysis. The data is used to better predict and manage illnesses and diseases. The software is also used to facilitate care delivery across populations based on need. In some ways, it caters to clusters of people, but it ultimately helps improve the quality of individualized patient care. After all, the analysis of population data leads to better prediction of individual health risks and a more accurate big-picture representation of health trends within different communities.

Hospitals and associated clinics have turned to AI solutions over the course of the pandemic to improve resource efficiency, strengthen diagnostics, and manage patient volumes. This is particularly critical in preventive care, especially with orthopedic surgery. Orthopedic surgeries are expected to rise from 22.3 million in 2017 to 28.3 million in 2022 worldwide. When factoring in the scarcity of resources, that places pressure on surgeons, clinicians, radiologists and all other medical specialists.

Deep learning–based technologies, like Zebra Medical Vision, ease the burden by providing radiologists with medical imaging analytics for scans and automatically analyzing them for various clinical findings. Such findings can be passed onto doctors, who can take the reports into consideration when making a diagnosis.[3, 4]

Looking at the intersection of population health management and healthcare data analytics could be interesting, as each market is set to become a $40 billion market within a couple of years. If we're examining the genomic space alone, the tipping point is around the corner with an affordable cost of $600 for full genome sequencing today, on track for $100 sequencing in just a few years. As genomic data becomes financially plausible and the data generated from genomics doubles every year, expected to reach 20 exabytes by 2025, the 5,000 geneticists worldwide won't be able to process a significant fraction of it. Healthcare data analytics in population health will be essential.

Precision medicine must rely on proper data processing and analysis. The AI models are already powerful enough—they just need the data to work with. Genetic-interpretation company Emedgene developed the concept of cognitive genomic intelligence—an inclusive, ever-growing platform that automatically produces insights from genomic data, reducing the time and cost of its interpretation, which traditionally requires hours of manual review and yields limited insights when solely relying on human intelligence.

H2O.AI is another solution that uses AI to analyze data throughout healthcare systems to mine, automate, and predict processes. The ever-popular IBM Watson Health uses AI to provide value-based care solutions for population health management, directly benefiting providers, health plans, employers, and pharmaceutical and biotech organizations.

16.4   Is Health Tech the New Healthcare?

Health Tech is the fastest-growing discipline within the healthcare sector. It includes any technology-enabled healthcare product and service that can be delivered or consumed outside of a hospital or physician's office.[5]

One notable exception is hospital and practice management software.

I was looking for a definition of *Health Tech* and found this graph (Figure 16.1) that maybe could help or clarify the concept. A clear definition

Content of Health Tech:

Health Tech	Robotics, nanotech, wearables, biosensors, 3D printing, Internet of Things (IoT), next-generation sequencing
Digital Health	Machine learning, AI, smart devices, big data, blockchain, apps
Healthcare IT	Software, electronic records, data security
Med Tech	Devices and software

Figure 16.1   Table of the different techniques in building health tech, digital health, healthcare IT, and MedTech.

of *Health Tech* seems to be hard to find. This is less optimal, as this leaves the concept to be unclear and, hence, open for misinterpretation.

16.5 Can Technology Help?

There are numerous problems with the healthcare environment, but the most challenging parts are supply and demand. The demand for healthcare is much higher than the supply, and it will continue to be a major challenge. The existing deficit of doctors and nurses will most likely get worse in the future. In some cities and at some times, there is also a shortage of hospital beds and medical devices. Medical devices and prescriptions are costly to develop and produce. Our healthcare demand is dramatically increasing as the population ages and, of course, as we deal with global health crises. Technology is critical to help overcome the supply and demand problem.

Technology can and will have a significant and positive effect on our lives in numerous ways. It can significantly reduce healthcare costs, improve patient access, and improve healthcare and associated diagnoses. Everything from telehealth, to online medical records, to the exciting new uses of AI can save money and increase health and well-being.

16.6 Telehealth

Telehealth saves over 100 minutes of patients' time compared to an in-person visit, according to an American investigation. They can conduct each appointment anywhere in the world where there's a telephone or internet connection. This time can be directly applied back into a productive workday or to increase an employee's quality of life. For several technologies and health and wellness companies, telehealth represents a vast, mostly untapped market. For all employees, telehealth enables increases in the company's bottom line and improvements in employee health and well-being.

About 90% of US healthcare providers had full-functioning or were developing telehealth programs before 2020. Then in the first half of 2020, patient adoption of telehealth services grew by 33% over the previous year. The estimate is that telehealth funding could reach $185 billion by 2026. Employers could save up to $6 billion per year on healthcare costs by providing telemedicine technologies to their employees. In one study of cardiovascular patients, telehealth options reduce the patient's monthly healthcare costs by $576.

It is incredible just how much virtual care can accomplish. It currently extends well beyond general medical and mental healthcare services. For example, one provider, Teladoc Health, provides direct-to-consumer services, platforms that support the physician practice, and platforms and models that help hospitals and health systems with everything from tele-ICU, tele-stroke, and tele-neonatal care. Teladoc Health was able to help reestablish an entire practice, Paradise Medical Group, after the California wildfires destroyed all its facilities.

Patients can send doctors a message online. The nurse can triage the questions and have the doctor answer the questions as needed when it is convenient for the doctor. The patient does not have to wait on hold or make an unnecessary appointment, which costs, on average, $150 per visit with insurance. Telehealth increases the number of patients healthcare providers can see while also improving patient access to valuable health information, which could reduce the cost substantially but also improve healthcare if we are able to quickly and effectively get our healthcare questions answered by a healthcare provider instead of Dr. Google. Telehealth visits are likely to speed up the initial stages of doctor and nurse consultancies compared to traditional, in-person visits we are used to presently.

The simple process of making healthcare more accessible increases patients' engagement with their health and increases the accuracy of diagnoses.

16.7   Other Healthcare Technologies of High Importance

If a healthcare provider has the right technology, they can store patient information in the cloud under safe conditions. Access to data improves diagnoses because all information is available for all providers that a patient sees. The data can then enable AI and other forms of predictive analytics to help the patient's condition and therapy.

Like so many parts of our lives now, technology advances that once seemed far away or impossible now exist. With the correct information, AI can learn about a patient's health by looking for trends and patterns. Google and another good example of the new modern trends is how Apple has been using GPS during the past several months to see where people have been and track if people have entered high-risk areas or been in contact with infected people during the pandemic.

Technology can so dramatically improve our lives, and healthcare has been one area that is rather slow to adapt to changes.

Regulations and privacy concerns are two primary factors that have caused the delays. The global health crisis with the Covid-19 pandemic has pushed us to embrace health technologies in new ways, and now, we are seeing other benefits. The new technology could also lead to bringing doctors the benefit of greater convenience and flexibility with the ability to work anytime and anywhere. It should also significantly reduce some of the healthcare costs.

16.8   Five Different Technological Innovations Changing Medical Practice

With technology, the past decade has been a revelation. Tech developers are breaking new ground, doing what we once thought was impossible. For engineers, researchers, and developers, it seems the question to ask now is not if it can be done but how.

Virtually every sector of the economy is experiencing the refreshing impact of technological innovation. Particularly in the health sector, there are plenty of business opportunities for entrepreneurs and investors.

Later, you will see descriptions of some of the hottest areas of the industry.

16.8.1   Robot-Assisted Surgery

This is often a mix of a sophisticated robotic surgical system and the special skills of highly trained surgeons. It is usually adopted for minimally invasive surgery. That is, where tiny incisions are made within the body and a laparoscopic machine is inserted into the opening. The machine includes a high-resolution camera, which captures the insides of the patient in 3D and guides the movements of the surgeon. The photographs from the camera are then magnified to permit the surgeon to make elaborate movements in tiny spaces.

While this innovation at this stage will cost more, it comes with notable benefits for the patient. The patient would have fewer scars, experience far less pain, and only spend a few days in the hospital, as the recovery time is usually shorter. For the doctor, they can operate with more precision and vision. Overall, robot-assisted surgery is beneficial to everyone involved, and it's becoming increasingly preferred among individuals who go under the knife.

16.8.2   Telemedicine

A few years back, it might have been difficult to imagine seeing a doctor without being in the same room together with the doctor. Those days, one had to wait in long queues even if only to get a quick consultation.

But with the presence of advanced communication technology, a wide range of online multimedia platforms, and even virtual reality, individuals can get healthcare wherever and whenever they need it.

Someone could be seeking guidance on symptoms they're having, and they can get answers right from their phone or laptop screen without ever visiting the hospital. Telemedicine is also helping to bridge the gap between medical practitioners in developed nations and people in third-world countries where healthcare structures are often quite poor.

The reliability of secure multimedia communications, coupled with precision devices able to transmit real-time data, is changing the landscape of the clinician–patient relationship such that standards of care do not de facto rely solely on office visits. These changes are made realistic due to rapid technological developments.

The Covid-19 pandemic forced us to improve digital technology, and many new technologies have been developed very fast, and these technologies have increased the speed with the introduction into the healthcare sector.

16.8.3   Nanomedicine

The smaller the better. Computer manufacturing companies and other makers of tech hardware strive to make their products as light and small as possible, without compromising quality and user satisfaction. That design philosophy is coming to a hospital near you soon and not just for aesthetics.

Patients can now have inserted microscopic devices into their bodies to get diagnoses. A few years ago, an Israeli company began developing a pill camera that can be used to monitor the large intestine and detect polyps as well as early signs of cancer in individuals.

Today, this technology has been accepted in close to 100 countries and is in high demand.

16.8.4   Artificial Intelligence

The intelligence of machines and software offers limitless possibilities for medical practice. AI algorithms can be employed to emulate human knowledge within the analysis of complex medical data. It can be used for diagnosis and predictions based on its own logic.

With AI, it is expected that performance and productivity will be optimized, and waste brought to a bare minimum. This will improve overall efficiency in the healthcare delivery sector. When applied to big data from across various sectors, helpful insights can be derived on several issues, such as predicting the spread of pandemics or deducing a cure for a disease based on cell therapy, which is what we are pioneering in the fight against multiple sclerosis. According to Sergey L. Mikheev, MD, CEO of Swiss Medica, artificial intelligence (AI) has disrupted numerous industries:

> Healthcare has flourished because of AI, even before the pandemic, as machine intelligence makes scanning large populations for diseases feasible and drives a proactive approach to healthcare—keeping people healthy instead of waiting for them to get sick.

As the name suggests, *population health* focuses on cohorts over individuals. For researchers in healthcare, population health relies on keeping track of the incidence of diseases in a variety of groups of people. For example, they could compare Covid-19 outbreaks among individuals of different demographics who reside in a range of ZIP codes. It focuses on the prevention or early detection of disease in large populations through screening.

This is different from the more generalized public health, which examines the health condition of a whole population of individuals. Public health calls for an analysis of pollutants in the air and water. Tending to population health requires the examination of disease incidence in groups according to criteria such as age, gender, or location.

16.8.5   Medical Chain

Another interesting technology the health sector is leveraging is blockchain. Recently, a major American healthcare provider, the Mayo Clinic, collaborated with a UK-based blockchain company for the deployment of an open and decentralized Medicare platform that keeps a patient in control of their personal data.

This platform is used to link patients with researchers and pharmaceutical companies, manage health records, and improve the security of data, thereby bolstering the trust of patients in the healthcare system. Blockchain also holds limitless possibilities for the healthcare sector, including financial and other sectors.

Most of these technological innovations are not futuristic; they are already being used to boost productivity and improve overall performance in medical practice.

16.9   Advanced Precision Medicine

Healthcare tailored specifically for you. Precision medicine is a product of our digital world—one in which genetic testing is now available and wearable technology, like Fitbits, can read vital signs in a flash. The ready availability of this kind of health data enables providers to create customized treatment plans suited to everyone. Patients are experiencing the wonders of such precision medicine in the form of immunotherapy for cancer as well as drugs specially formulated for cystic fibrosis patients with a particular gene mutation. Further, those who need medical devices are increasingly able to get them individually designed and sized, thanks to digital imaging and 3D printing.

Increased adoption of AI is only accelerating these advances in precision medicine.[6]

Reference List, Chapter 16

1 Prof. Borlak, Fraunhofer Institute, Hannover, Germany, Personal communications, Approx. 2011
2 www.zebra.com/gb/en.html
3 www.nanox.vision/ai
4 www.linkedin.com/pulse/what-healthtech-jorge-juan-fernández-garc%C3%ADa?trk= public_profile_article_view https://es.linkedin.com/in/jorgejuanfernandez?trk= pulse-article_main-author-card
5 www.brookings.edu/research/advancing-precision-medicine-through-agile-governance/
6 https://www.ncbi.nlm.nih.gov/pmc/articles/PMC7877825

17

AN INTRODUCTION TO THE CLINICAL CHAPTERS ON CANCER AND CARDIOVASCULAR AND NEUROLOGICAL DISEASES

The earlier two parts of this book (Chapters 1–15) have covered the history of our healthcare journey and the new inventions, showing how we were able to move from mystification and religion to a scientific approach with facts and clinical proof in order to cure sick people, which has led to increasing the life expectancy continuously from 25–30 years to 90 years or, soon, even 100 years. As I have mentioned, maybe the first persons to reach 130 years of age have already been born. This is a remarkable development.

Note: In May 2022, we read in newspapers that a woman died at the age of 119 years. Therefore, it is reasonable to guess that we are on the way to reaching the 130-year threshold, within a reasonable time frame.

In this part of the book, we will look at the different, new, and ongoing research and developments that may reach the market and a larger population, looking at 2050 and beyond. We will start with an overview of what we can diagnose and to what extent we can treat diseases in three different categories: cancers, cardiovascular diseases, and neurological diseases.

17.1 Confronting the Big 6 Health Issues (Excluding Pathogens)

The six most devasting diseases seen from a population point of view are as follows:

- Cardiac/cardiovascular disease
- Breast cancer
- Alzheimer's disease
- Diabetes
- Colon cancer
- Lung cancer

The way we are approaching and attacking these six healthcare issues that are so devastating to individuals who get the diseases as well as for our societies as a whole, thinking about the resources, costs, and lives that are wasted are

DOI: 10.1201/9781003393320-21

listed as follows. Our approach to standing up against these diseases can be outlined in the following ways. Actions to conquer the diseases are as follows:

- Finding the diseases earlier; in reality, before we have symptoms and before we can feel or sense anything of the diseases.
- Integrating biology, chemistry, physics, engineering, genomics, and information. We are not there yet but working on it.

To me, this means a lot of integrated research must be pursued in combination with an integrated clinical approach and a clear strategic plan in order to become successful.

17.1.1   Reminder

When we discuss diseases and healthcare in general, we are in the field of applied science. We must not forget that before we are able to reach the stage of applied science, there are, almost all the time, many years of basic research being pursued where proof of principles for specific methods are developed, evaluated, and validated. This involves an in-depth understanding of a specific human organ and its detailed function. The time it takes to introduce a new product or procedure into the healthcare system is also a time-consuming process.

All this is needed in order to continue to build the evidence-based medicine we want as the foundation of our modern healthcare.

17.1.2   The Need for Basic Scientific Research in an Applied Age

A good foundation is critical to the stability of any structure. The same could be said for the real-world application of scientific discoveries. Before any new idea can be applied outside the lab, it needs to go through a process that starts with an idea or discovery. Then, through in-depth research and iterative improvements, a viable product can be developed, whether it be a new disease treatment or a new, faster computer method.

Applied science would never work as a stand-alone research field. It needs to be based on a strong basic science foundation.

This type of basic research strengthens the work at South Korea's Pohang University of Science and Technology (POSTECH). There, researchers embrace the fundamentals of their work to gain a deeper understanding of the problem under investigation, while also being encouraged to collaborate across disciplines to nurture more innovative solutions. This leads to more robust applied research and higher-quality outcomes.[1-3]

17.2   We Are Entering a New Era in Healthcare

The handling and curing of acutely and severely sick people will continue with gradually improved knowledge and new developments and techniques sometimes with smaller incremental steps and, occasionally, with more dramatic changes, what I have called quantum leaps.

We will also be able to find new risk factors and biomarkers with the possibility to start diagnostics and treatments earlier and, hopefully, before symptoms are recognized.

With the possibility of such dramatic changes, many new challenges will also follow.

17.2.1   Many Diseases, One Answer?

"When it comes to treating most diseases, immunotherapy will be the answer," says Gary K. Michelson. An interesting statement that can and should probably be challenged?[4]

17.3   The New, Modern Swiss Army Knife: Our Beloved Smartphone

We all know that if you have a Swiss Army knife in your pocket, your chances of getting out of a challenging or even threatening situation increase when you are trespassing or hiking. Today, there is a new thing that almost none of us leave more than an arm's length from ourselves, the mobile phone.

Well, it is not so new anymore, but it becomes more and more capable and, therefore, almost indispensable for us all.

Many of the features, besides making phone calls, are linked to commercial activities, but there are also many new possibilities and ideas that are linked to our healthcare that will continue and expand looking forward. The name *mobile phone* is almost becoming obsolete, as making phone calls is almost an understatement of what mobiles can do today.

I remember the times when we installed the transportable mobile battery pack in the rear of our car and then took the headset or microphone and installed this in the front so we could answer when driving. It was probably the late 1980s or maybe at the beginning of the 1990s. It was a fantastic feeling to become so connected.[5]

Personal Anecdote

During my time as the technical manager for GE Medical Systems Sweden, I had the pleasure of being able to introduce mobile phones to my engineers. Everybody on the team was very happy, as it saved the engineers a lot of travel up and down in the long country of Sweden (in fact, 2,500 km from south to the very north). My boss in the UK was, on the contrary, very unhappy, as he felt we had set a precedence for his engineer to request mobile phones. I was called to London to explain the advantages for Sweden and motivate his engineers not to request the same. This was during the time we used overheads. I had prepared overhead slides. One with the map of Sweden, and one with the map of the UK with the same scale. So I started presenting our case and how much we saved in travel time. Then I flipped the map of the UK onto the Swedish map, and the UK reached half the length of Sweden.

Everyone thought it was a great and convincing case. My boss was happy for the moment. The following year, mobile phones for all engineers were budgeted. Now, everybody was happy! The service level both in Sweden and the UK was improved very much.

17.3.1 Medical Examples Where the Smartphone Is Being Used Today

17.3.1.1 Administration of Insulin for Diabetics

The Food and Drug Administration cleared the first app for iPhone and Android devices capable of giving diabetes patients doses of insulin.

In a statement, Tandem Diabetes Care confirmed its connect mobile app, which pairs with the company's t:slim.X2 insulin pump, will allow diabetic users to administer a dose of insulin directly through their smartphone. The feature is used for bolus insulin dosing, said the company. According to the nonprofit organization Beyond Type 1, bolus insulin is a type of insulin taken to prevent glucose spikes after meals.

"This FDA clearance further validates our commitment to innovation and the diabetes community by providing one of the most requested feature enhancements," said John Sheridan, president and CEO of Tandem Diabetes Care.

There are many more and a continuous and steadily growing number of examples of new apps and new technology developments that use and will use our mobile phone as the hub and gather information from a sensor or similar inputs, like heart rate and atrial fibrillation.[8]

Nobody is capable of predicting the breakthroughs in technology that will happen in the future

Nobody knew in 1980 that in 2008, we all would be carrying an advanced computer in our pocket or that each one of us would be able to communicate with everyone in the whole world in real time.

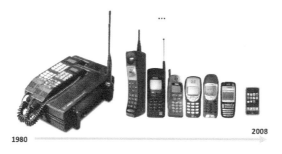

We don't know what we don't know until afterward; then we all know!

Figure 17.1 The development of the transportable phone into a portable advanced communication device. (Unknown source)[6, 7]

Reference List, Chapter 17

1 https://en.wikipedia.org/wiki/Pohang_University_of_Science_and_Technology
2 www.indeed.com/career-advice/career-development/basic-research-vs-applied-research
3 https://international.postech.ac.kr
4 www.cancer.org/treatment/treatments-and-side-effects/treatment-types/immuno-therapy.html
5 https://digitalhealth.modernhealthcare.com/technology/will-your-smartphone-be-next-doctors-office
6 Unknown Source: The Development of the Transportable Phone into a Portable Advanced Communication Device
7 www.sciencemuseum.org.uk/objects-and-stories/invention-mobile-phones
8 www.ncbi.nlm.nih.gov/pmc/articles/PMC3510747/

18

PRESENT STATUS OF CANCER IN THE YEAR 2022

18.1 The Definition of Cancer

Cancer is caused by changes (mutations) to the DNA within cells. The DNA inside a cell is packaged into many individual genes, each of which contains a set of instructions telling the cell what functions to perform as well as how to grow and divide.

Cancer is a disease in which some of the body's cells grow uncontrollably and spread to other parts of the body. Cancer can start almost anywhere in the human body, which is made up of trillions of cells. Normally, human cells grow and multiply (through a process called cell division) to form new cells as the body needs them. When cells grow old or become damaged, they die, and new cells take their place.

Sometimes, this orderly process breaks down, and abnormal or damaged cells grow and multiply when they shouldn't. These cells may form tumors, which are lumps of tissue. Tumors can be cancerous or not cancerous (benign).

Cancerous tumors spread into, or invade, nearby tissues and can travel to distant places in the body to form new tumors (a process called metastasis). Cancerous tumors are also called malignant tumors. Many cancers form solid tumors, but cancers of the blood, such as leukemias, generally do not.

Benign tumors do not spread into, or invade, nearby tissues. When removed, benign tumors usually don't grow back, whereas cancerous tumors sometimes do. Benign tumors can sometimes be quite large, however. Some can cause serious symptoms or be life-threatening, such as benign tumors in the brain.

Cancer is a disease in which some of the body's cells grow uncontrollably and spread to other parts of the body. Cancer can start almost anywhere in the human body, which is made up of trillions of cells.[1]

There Are Four Major Categories of Cancer

1. *Carcinomas*: Most common, epithelial tissue.
2. *Sarcomas*: Tumors made of connective tissue cells.
3. *Lymphomas*: (a) Affect cells involved in the immune system and (b) Hodgkin's disease.
4. *Leukemias*: Cancer of blood-forming parts of the bone (bone marrow).[2, 3]

DOI: 10.1201/9781003393320-22

Risk Factors for Getting Cancer

- Smoking
- Heavy alcohol consumption
- Excess body weight
- Physical inactivity
- Poor nutrition

Currently, the most significant unpreventable risk factor is age. According to the American Cancer Society, doctors in the United States diagnose 87% of cancer cases in people of ages 50 years or older.[4, 5]

There is consistent evidence that men are more likely to get cancer and die from it compared to women. According to the Canadian Cancer Society, the lifetime probability of developing cancer is 49% for men and 45% for women, and the probability of dying from cancer is 28% for men and 24% for women.

18.1.1   How Prevalent Is Cancer Today?

According to one study published in *JAMA Oncology*, and based on data from the Global Burden of Diseases, Injuries, and Risk Factors Study, 2019, 18.7 million people worldwide received a cancer diagnosis in 2010, and the total deaths from cancer numbered 8.29 million.

In 2019, those numbers had increased significantly, with 23.6 million people receiving a new cancer diagnosis and records documenting 10 million cancer deaths.

The scientists who conducted the research also found that among 22 groups of injuries and diseases studied, cancer was the second leading cause of death, years of life lost, and disability-adjusted life years.

The World Health Organization (WHO) indicates that the most common types of cancers diagnosed in 2020 were as follows:

- Breast cancer (2.26 million diagnoses)
- Lung cancer (2.21 million diagnoses)
- Colon and rectal cancer (1.93 million diagnoses)
- Prostate cancer (1.41 million diagnoses)
- Nonmelanoma skin cancer (1.20 million diagnoses)
- Stomach cancer (1.09 million diagnoses)

The deaths for each cancer category in 2020 were as follows:

- Lung cancer, caused 1.8 million deaths
- Colorectal cancer, caused 935,000 deaths
- Liver cancer, 830,000 deaths
- Stomach cancer, 769,000 deaths
- Breast cancer, 685,000 deaths

As mentioned earlier, statistics indicate that males experience a higher cancer mortality rate than females. Additionally, the death rate from cancer is highest among Black males and lowest among Asian and Pacific Islander females.

Despite these statistics, the American Cancer Society suggests that, in the United States, the overall cancer mortality rate has been steadily decreasing over the last 28 years.

The organization indicates the death rate from cancer fell by 32% between 1991 and 2019 when considering data from males and females.

Factors that may play a role in this decrease include the following:

- A reduction in the number of people who smoke, as smoking is the leading cause of lung cancer.
- The addition of chemotherapy treatment after surgery for breast and colon cancer, and the use of combination therapy for many cancers.
- The advancement of prevention and early detection strategies for some cancer types.

Progress with diagnosing lung cancer in the localized stage and improvements in surgical techniques and treatment medications may play a role in the improved survival rate.

18.1.2　What Forms of Cancer Are on the Rise?

Although the overall mortality rate from cancer may be decreasing, certain types of cancer are on the rise. For example, according to Cancer Statistics, 2022, published in the American Cancer Society's journal, *CA*.

In *Cancer Journal for Clinicians*, data from 2014 to 2018 indicated a 0.5% annual increase in female breast cancer. At the same time, the incidence of prostate cancer remained stable.

Between 2015 and 2050, the Centers for Disease Control and Prevention (CDC), expects new cancer diagnoses in the United States to stabilize in females and decrease in males.

However, the CDC projects that colorectal, prostate, and female breast cancers will rise, and cancer diagnoses in older adults will increase due to an aging population. In addition, research indicates that from 1973 to 2015, certain subtypes of cancer—specifically carcinoma of the kidney—have risen in adolescents and young adults in the United States, with an overall cancer rate increase of 29.6% in this age group.

18.1.3　What Is Causing an Increase in Cancer Rates?

Although we are making progress with some types of cancer, the National Cancer Institute suggests that the incidence of other cancers may rise due to an increase in some risk factors.

These include the fact that people are living longer, as a person's cancer risk tends to increase as we grow older, and the fact that many people also suffer from obesity. Reports suggest that people with obesity may have an increased risk for certain types of cancer. Worldwide, 650 million adults were affected by obesity in 2016.

In addition, continued difficulties with accessing quality healthcare due to socioeconomic challenges or racial bias may contribute to an increase in cancer rates.

For example, according to a WHO report, 90% of countries in the high-income group have comprehensive treatment available. In comparison, less than 15% of countries in the low-income group have access to quality treatments.[6]

18.2   Diagnostic Methods for Detecting Cancers

Some examples are as follows.

18.2.1   Biopsy

Diagnostic procedures used to screen for diseases like cancer usually involve an analysis of tissue or blood, often from a biopsy.

During a biopsy, a doctor removes a sample of tissue or fluid from the body. A pathologist inspects the cells under a microscope to determine whether they are cancerous. If the cells are found to be cancerous, a biopsy may help determine whether cancer began at the site of the biopsy or if it started somewhere else in the body and spread to the biopsy site.

18.2.2   Bronchoscopy

Bronchoscopy is a procedure done to look inside the air passages of your lungs. In the most common type, flexible bronchoscopy, a thin and flexible scope is inserted through your nose or mouth. The scope, called a broncho-scope, is passed down the back of your throat and between your vocal cords to enter the air passages.

A camera in the scope sends pictures to a video screen during the procedure.

18.2.3   Endoscopy

Endoscopy is the umbrella term for a group of medical procedures that use an endoscope—a thin, tubular scope with a lens and light—to examine the inside of your body. This way, your doctor can see tissues inside the body closely to look for abnormal changes, blockages, growths, or other issues that may be causing symptoms.

In some cases, the scope also has a tool for the removal of tissue to be examined for disease.

18.2.4   Colonoscopy

This procedure is performed to examine the inside of the colon and rectum. It's performed with a type of endoscope called a colonoscope. The scope is inserted through the anus and into the rectum and colon. Additional instruments can be moved through the scope in order to take a biopsy or remove areas of tissue that look suspicious, such as polyps.

18.2.5   Cystoscopy

This procedure is performed to examine the inside of the bladder and urethra. It's performed with a type of endoscope called a cystoscope. The scope is inserted via the urethra, which carries urine to the outside of the body.

18.2.6   Laparoscopy

Laparoscopy, also known as keyhole surgery, is performed to examine the inside of the abdomen and pelvis. It's performed with a type of endoscope called a laparoscope. The scope is inserted via a small incision made in the abdominal wall near the belly button. Additional incisions may be made in other areas of the belly to insert additional instruments.

18.2.7   Laryngoscopy

This procedure is performed to examine the vocal cords, other structures of the larynx (voice box), and adjacent structures, such as the back of the throat.

18.2.8   Mediastinoscopy

This procedure is performed to examine the inside of the mediastinum, located between your lungs and the back of your breastbone. It's performed with a type of endoscope called a mediastinoscopy. The scope is inserted via a small incision right above the breastbone and slowly moved into the mediastinum.

18.2.9   Thoracoscopy

This procedure is performed to examine the area inside the chest and outside the lungs. It is performed with a type of endoscope called a thoracoscope. The scope is inserted through a small incision made near the lower section of the shoulder blade.

In some cases, thoracoscopy is performed as part of video-assisted thoracoscopic surgery, or VATS, a surgical procedure that allows your doctor to examine the inside of your lungs and chest cavity. It's used both for diagnosing and treating health issues within the lungs and chest.

18.2.10   Cytology Tests

A cytology test examines cells through body fluids and tissues. These tests may be used to look for cancer when a patient is due for regular screening or is experiencing symptoms.

18.2.11   Lumbar Puncture

A lumbar puncture, or spinal tap, is a procedure during which a needle is inserted into the lower part of the spinal column to remove a sample of cerebrospinal fluid. The fluid surrounds and protects the brain and spinal cord.

18.2.12   Pathology Reports

After a biopsy is collected, your tissue sample will be evaluated microscopically. These results—along with laboratory, imaging, and other diagnostic testing—are used to establish whether cancer is present, as well as the extent of the cancer, which helps determine treatment options.

18.2.13   Genetic Testing

Genetic testing is becoming more and more common in order to individualize cancer treatments.

Genetics is the study of the genes people inherit at birth, passed on from their family through the generations. Every cell in the human body has a complete strand of DNA, and each strand is packed with genes, which carry instructions for certain traits, such as blue eyes, red hair, or perhaps, a stronger likelihood of certain cancers. Genetic tests may help identify a person's risk of cancer and other diseases.

18.3   Medical Imaging Tools for Detecting Cancers

- Computerized tomography (CT) scanning
- Magnetic resonance imaging (MRI) scanning
- X-rays and other radiographic tests
- Mammography
- Nuclear medicine scans (bone scans, PET scans, thyroid scans, MUGA [multigated acquisition] scans, gallium scans)
- Ultrasound

18.4   Specific Diagnostic Imaging Tools for Cancer

We have today the capability to image most critical parameters that are needed in order to diagnose and follow-up on cancer development after treatment.

The following hallmarks of cancer can all be imaged today:

- *Lymph nodes*: https://en.wikipedia.org/wiki/Lymph_node
- *Amino acid metabolism*: https://en.wikipedia.org/wiki/Protein_metabolism
- *Hypoxia*: https://en.wikipedia.org/wiki/Hypoxia_(medical)
- *Angiogenesis*: https://en.wikipedia.org/wiki/Angiogenesis
- *Mitochondria function*: https://en.wikipedia.org/wiki/Mitochondrion
- *Proliferation*: https://en.wikipedia.org/wiki/Cell_proliferation

18.4.1   All the Earlier Parameters Can Be Imaged with PET, Some with MRI Techniques, and Some with SPECT

The imaging options in connection with cancer diagnostics have made tremendous progress over the last 20 years. From only being able to image the location and the morphology of cancer to being able to see the functionality and characterization of the cancer. This will enable an improved staging of cancer for improved treatments.

For most types of cancer, doctors need to know how much cancer there is and where it is (among other things) to help determine the best treatment options.

For example, the best treatment for early-stage cancer may be surgery or radiation, while a more advanced-stage cancer may need treatments that reach all parts of the body, such as chemotherapy, targeted drug therapy, or immunotherapy.

The stage of cancer is also a way for doctors to describe the extent of the cancer when they talk with each other about a person's cancer.[7]

Cancer research is making remarkable progress. Today, we know in rather detail what is happening when a normal cell is converting to a cancer cell.

If you received a cancer diagnosis 40–50 years ago, you would have had approximately a 60% risk of dying of the disease. Today, this risk is only around 30%.

The chances of surviving a cancer diagnosis are improving year by year.[8]

On September 12, 2022, American President Biden was in Boston, Massachusetts, reigniting Moonshot for Cancer under the leadership of the White House. The plan is to reduce cancer deaths by 50% within the coming 25 years and improve the experience of people and their families living with and surviving cancer and, by doing this and more, end cancer as we know it today. This is an ambitious plan, but it seems realistic to me with the massive progress we have made in the past 20 years.[9]

18.4.2   Therapeutic Tools That Are Used to Treat Cancer

- Surgery
- Chemotherapy
- Radiation therapy

- Targeted therapy
- Immunotherapy—checkpoint inhibitor
- Stem cell or bone marrow transplant
- Hormone therapy

Surgery is still the most common method of removing primary cancer tumors. Our challenge today is that in case the cancer has spread to other organs, the therapeutic procedure becomes very much more challenging or complicated.

Therefore, it is often said that the most important way to reduce the risk for the cancer patient is early detection, as this reduces the risk of discovering metastasis.

In many cases, surgery is not possible due to the cancer being too close to a specific organ or nerves with a high risk for the surgery itself to fail by hurting another organ.

Surgery is many times combined with chemotherapy. Chemotherapy can be used to shrink the tumor before surgery or after surgery in order to secure that all cancer cells are removed after treatment.[10]

18.5   Ongoing Interesting Research That Is Likely to Materialize in Clinical Procedures in the (Near) Future

1. **New technology could make biopsies a thing of the past** by Columbia University School of Engineering and Applied Science

A Columbia engineering team has developed a technology that could replace conventional biopsies and histology with real-time imaging within the living body. As described in a new paper published today in *Nature Biomedical Engineering*, MediSCAPE is a high-speed 3D microscope capable of capturing images of tissue structures that could guide surgeons to navigate tumors and their boundaries without needing to remove tissues and wait for pathology results.

For many medical procedures, particularly cancer surgery and screening, it is common for doctors to take a biopsy, cutting out small pieces of tissue to be able to take a closer look at them with a microscope.

> The way that biopsy samples are processed hasn't changed in 100 years, they are cut out, Sxed, embedded, sliced, stained with dyes, positioned on a glass slide, and viewed by a pathologist using a simple microscope. This is why it can take days to hear news back about your diagnosis after a biopsy.
>
> *Elizabeth Hillman, Professor of Biomedical Engineering and Radiology at Columbia University and Senior Author of the Study*

Hillman's group dreamed of a bold alternative, wondering whether they could capture images of the tissue while it is still within the body. "Such a technology could give a doctor real- time feedback about what type of tissue they are looking at without the long wait," she explains. "This instant answer would let them make informed decisions about how best to cut out a tumor and ensure there is none left behind."

Another major benefit of the approach is that cutting tissue out, just to figure out what it is, is a hard decision for doctors, especially for precious tissues, such as the brain, spinal cord, nerves, the eye, and areas of the face. This means that doctors can miss important areas of disease. "Because we can image the living tissue, without cutting it out, we hope that MediSCAPE will make those decisions a thing of the past," says Hillman.

2. **New 3D imaging method may help doctors better determine prostate cancer aggressiveness** by Sarah McQuate, University of Washington, December 9, 2021

A team led by the University of Washington has developed a new, non-destructive method of 3D biopsies instead of just a slice. Prostate cancer is the most common cancer for men, and for men in the United States, it's the second leading cause of death.

Some prostate cancers might be slow-growing and can be monitored over time, whereas others need to be treated right away. To determine how aggressive someone's cancer is, doctors look for abnormalities in slices of biopsied tissue on a slide. But this 2D method makes it hard to properly diagnose borderline cases.

Now a team led by the University of Washington has developed a new, non-destructive method that images entire 3D biopsies instead of just a slice. In a proof-of-principle experiment, the researchers imaged 300 3D biopsies taken from 50 patients—6 biopsies per patient—and had a computer use 3D and 2D results to predict the likelihood that a patient had aggressive cancer. The 3D features made it easier for the computer to identify the cases that were more likely to recur within five years.

The team published these results December 1, 2021, in *Cancer Research.*

> We show for the first time that compared to traditional pathology—where a small fraction of each biopsy is examined in 2D on microscope slides—the ability to examine 100% of a biopsy in 3D is more informative and accurate.
>
> This is exciting because it is the first of hopefully many clinical studies that will demonstrate the value of non-destructive 3D pathology for clinical decision-making, such as determining which patients require aggressive treatments or which subsets of patients would respond best to certain drugs.
>
> *Senior Author Jonathan Liu, a UW Professor of*
> *Mechanical Engineering and Bioengineering*

The researchers used prostate specimens from patients who underwent surgery more than 10 years ago, so the team knew each patient's outcome and could use that information to train a computer to predict those outcomes. In this study, half of the samples contained a more aggressive cancer.

3.   **Cause of metastasis in prostate cancer discovered** by Johannes Angerer, Medical University of Vienna, April 4, 2022

Prostate cancers remain localized in most cases, giving affected individuals a good chance of survival. However, about 20% of patients develop incurable metastatic prostate cancer, resulting in approximately 5,000 deaths each year in Austria alone. Medical research has not yet adequately explained why metastases occur in some people and not in others. A research team at MedUni Vienna has now discovered significant changes in a protein that drives the growth and spread of prostate cancer. The study was recently published in *Molecular Cancer*.

In the study, the researchers broke new ground and investigated the role of the protein KMT2C in prostate cancer. KMT2C is a genetic component that essentially functions as a regulator of central cellular processes. If KMT2C loses this regulatory ability due to typical cancer-related mutations, this encourages the proliferation of the cancer gene MYC. This in turn causes cells to divide at an increased rate, driving both the growth and spread of the cancer.

New insights into the transition to metastasis: "Our study provides new insights into the previously poorly understood transition from localized prostate cancer to terminal metastatic prostate cancer," says study leader Lukas Kenner (Department of Pathology at MedUni Vienna, Comprehensive Cancer Center of MedUni Vienna, and University Hospital Vienna, Department of Laboratory Animal Pathology at Vetmeduni Vienna, and the K1 Center CBmed), underlining the significance of the research work. In addition, the knowledge gained about the effects of KMT2C mutations may also generate new momentum for the diagnosis and treatment of prostate cancer.

Diagnosing aggressive progression at an early stage: KMT2C mutation status can be measured via a blood test, allowing early diagnosis of potentially aggressive progression in prostate cancers. In addition, MYC inhibitors could be used to prevent increased cell division, and hence, metastasis, and it is hoped that further scientific studies will substantiate this. MYC inhibitors are essentially new cancer treatment drugs that have already been tested in clinical trials and—if further studies confirm this—could also be used in metastatic prostate cancer in the next few years.

Since a high level of KMT2C mutation characterizes many types of cancer, such as breast, lung, colorectal, bladder and even skin cancer, our study results have a great deal of potential in the research, diagnosis and treatment of malignant cancers in general.

Lukas Kenner

4. **Researchers load CAR-T cells with oncolytic virus to treat solid cancer tumors** by Mayo Clinic, April 13, 2022

Researchers at Mayo Clinic's Center for Individualized Medicine have devised an immunotherapy technique that combines chimeric antigen receptor-T cell therapy, or CAR-T cell therapy, with a cancer-killing virus to target and treat solid cancer tumors more effectively. The combination approach, published in *Science Translational Medicine*, involves loading CAR-T cells, which are engineered to look for antigens on cancer cells, with an oncolytic virus. Oncolytic viruses are naturally occurring viruses that can infect and break down cancer cells. They either naturally replicate well in cancer cells or can be engineered to selectively target cancer cells. The study suggests CAR-T cells can deliver the oncolytic virus to the tumor. Then the virus can infiltrate tumor cells, replicate to bust the cells open, and stimulate a potent immune response. "This approach allows the tumor to be killed by the virus as well as by the CAR-T cells," explains Richard Vile, PhD, co-leader of the Gene and Virus Therapy Program within Mayo Clinic Cancer Center. "In addition, when the virus is delivered, it turns the tumor into a very inflammatory environment, which the patient's own immune system then sees and starts to attack."

The therapeutic strategy addresses two major challenges that make solid tumors difficult to treat with CAR-T cell therapy alone. First, the oncolytic virus can break down the molecular shield that some solid tumors use to avoid an immune system attack. Second, the virus can invade into the core of the cancer cells—a near-impossible feat for immune cells alone, which often lose their power in the attempt. The researchers also found that the combination approach provided an immune memory phenotype against the tumor. "By putting the virus onto the CAR-T, we activate them against both the virus and the tumor, and they acquire immunological memory," Dr. Vile says. "This allows us to give a boost with the virus at a later time point, which in turn makes the CAR-T cells wake up again and undergo additional rounds of killing the tumor."

5. **A new AI-powered X-ray technique for detecting explosives could identify cancer** Partridge, T., Astolfo, A., Shankar, S.S. et al. Enhanced detection of threat materials by dark-field x-ray imaging combined with deep neural networks. Nat Commun 13, 4651 (2022). https://doi.org/10.1038/s41467-022-32402-0. September 9, 2022

X-ray imaging has been boosted by the introduction of phase-based methods. Detail visibility is enhanced in phase contrast images, and dark-field images are sensitive to inhomogeneities on a length scale below the system's spatial resolution. Here, we show that the dark field creates a texture that is characteristic of the imaged material and that its combination with conventional attenuation leads to improved discrimination of threat materials. We show that the remaining ambiguities can be resolved by exploiting the different energy dependence of the dark field and attenuation signals. Furthermore, we demonstrate that the dark-field texture is well-suited for identification through machine learning approaches through two proof-of-concept studies. In both cases, the application of the same approaches to datasets from which the dark-field images were removed led to a clear degradation in performance. While the small scale of these studies means further research is required, results indicate a potential for combined use of dark-field and deep neural networks in security applications and beyond.

This is an interesting technique that could also be used in medical applications. The most interesting one is cancer detection at an early state.

6. A new approach to therapy-resistant tumors targets a specific cell-death pathway[11]

In a paper appearing in *Nature*, an international group of scientists report a new way to kill hard-to-treat cancers. These tumors resist current immunotherapies, including those using Nobel Prize–winning checkpoint-blocking antibodies.

The approach exploits Z-DNA. Rather than twisting to the right like B-DNA, Z-DNA has a left-handed twist. One role of Z-DNA is to regulate the immune response to viruses. The response involves AADR1 and ZBP1, two proteins that specifically recognize Z-DNA. They do so through a Zα domain that binds to the Z-DNA structure with high affinity.

The Zα domain was originally discovered by Dr. Alan Herbert of InsideOutBio, a communicating author on the paper. The ADAR1 Zα domain turns off the autoimmune response, while the other ZBP1 Zα turns on pathways that kill virally infected cells, as previously shown by Dr. Sid Balachandran, the other communicating author on the paper. The interactions between ADAR1 and ZBP1 determine whether a tumor cell lives or dies.

Both Zα proteins are induced by interferon during inflammation. They are not usually present in normal cells. Both proteins are also expressed in tumors, especially in normal cells called fibroblasts that cancer cells force to support their growth. Normally, tumors rely on ADAR1 to suppress cell death pathways that would otherwise kill the tumor.

The team found a small molecule that could bypass ADAR1 suppression and directly activate tumor cell death by ZBP1. The drug acts regardless of the mutation that causes the cancer. The form of cell death induced is highly immunogenic. The response destroys the fibroblasts supporting the tumor growth. By doing so, the drug enhances the effectiveness of immunotherapy using the checkpoint-blocking antibody targeted at PD-1. The drug is a member of the Curaxin family and was introduced to the clinic for another purpose. The compound has proven safe in Phase I trials but still requires further research to confirm its clinical use in conjunction with anti-PD1 provides a benefit in the treatment of cancers.

Dr. Herbert says as follows:

> this outcome is the work of a highly collaborative team. It is a nice milestone in our understanding of how alternative DNA conformations, like Z-DNA, play an important role in human biology. The paper shows how basic research can lead to new and unexpected therapies. The process has taken a long time, starting with the initial discovery of the Zα domain and then to the identification of Zα DNA variants that cause genetic diseases in humans. These discoveries validated a biological role for Z-DNA.
>
> The work has now led us to a new therapeutic approach for the treatment of cancer. It is a pleasing turnaround, given that the initial Z-DNA discoveries were widely dismissed by the scientific community as of little biological importance and further work was not ranked as worthy of funding by the National Institutes of Health peer review panels.

Z-DNA is formed in normal cells by sequences called flipons that, under physiological conditions, can reversibly flip to the left-handed conformation. The structure was discovered by accident in the first-ever synthetic crystal ever solved by X-ray crystallography. Other classes of flipons exist and are also highly likely to play important roles in biology. Flipons are highly dynamic structures that have been hard to study, as it is challenging to determine their exact conformation inside cells. Dr. Herbert says that "it is similar to other highly dynamic systems in physics where you can only find the flip on conformation by making a direct measurement, but only if the act of measurement does not bias the result."

7. Angiogenesis, cell signaling technology

Angiogenesis is defined as the physiological process by which new blood vessels are formed from pre-existing blood vessels. It is a critical process that enables development, skeletal muscle hypertrophy, menstruation, pregnancy, and wound healing, but it also contributes to pathological conditions, including neovascular disorders (retinopathy), rheumatoid arthritis, psoriasis, AIDS/Kaposi's sarcoma, and cancer (tumorigenesis). Angiogenesis is a complex and highly ordered process that relies upon extensive signaling networks both among and within endothelial cells (ESC), their associated mural cells (vascular smooth muscle cells [VSMCs] and pericytes), and other cell types (like immune cells).

Vascular endothelial growth factor (VEGF) is a family of proteins that are required for angiogenesis. There are multiple isoforms of VEGF, including VEGF-A, VEGF-B, VEGF-C, and VEGF-D, each playing a major role in different angiogenic contexts ranging from embryonic to lymphatic angiogenesis. VEGF-A is the principal mediator of angiogenesis. Alternative splicing produces four main VEGF-A isoforms of different lengths—121, 165, 189, and 206 amino acids long—which display varying affinities for heparan sulfate proteoglycans (HSPG). The balance between freely diffusible and HSPG-bound VEGF-A results in a gradient, leading to the formation of a pioneering tip cell—an endothelial cell that responds to angiogenic signaling. The tip cell creates the leading edge of the angiogenic sprout and, eventually, vascular branching through various steps of cell migration. The branches first expand with site-specific metabolic demands and are then subdivided into arteries, capillaries, veins, and lymphatic vessels, a process mediated by the Notch-Gridlock, Ephrin-B2/EphB4, and Sonic Hedgehog (SHH) pathways. With further vessel maturation and hemodynamic changes, ECs secrete platelet-derived growth factor (PDGF)-B to recruit pericytes and VSMCs. These mural cells, via expression of angiopoietin-1 (ANG-1), bind to ECs, resulting in TGF-β activation and extracellular matrix (ECM) deposition, thereby stabilizing the growing vascular bed. Downstream effectors—including phosphatidylinositol-3 kinase (PI3K), Src kinase, focal adhesion kinase (FAK), p38 mitogen-activated protein kinase (p38 MAPK), Smad2/3, and phospholipase C gamma (PLCγ)/Erk1/2—promote EC survival, vascular permeability, and migratory/proliferative phenotypes. Positive and negative transcriptional regulation of these moieties via microRNAs (miRNAs) further influence postnatal angiogenesis. Specifically, miR-126 has been shown to play a vital role, as deletion leads to defective vessel formation and embryonic lethality.

Pathological and physiological angiogenesis share many similarities in terms of signaling events and the resulting changes to cell function and behavior and, therefore, may be novel therapeutic options to combat disease. However, a key difference is that pathological vessel development is not terminated upon adequate tissue perfusion. Such uncontrolled, disorganized, unresolved growth precludes the advancement of novel angiogenesis-disrupting agents.[12]

8. Biomarker candidates for tumors identified from deep-profiled plasma stem

Proteins control most biological processes in life. Alterations in their expression level, localization, and proteoforms are often correlated with disease onset and progression. (1) In humans and animals, blood flows through virtually all tissues. Therefore, it has the potential to indicate the health state of any inner organ, even those not accessible from the outside. Blood is readily obtainable with minimal invasive sampling, and large biobanks exist for retrospective analyses. (2) Clinical analysis of blood is the most widespread diagnostic procedure in medicine, and blood biomarkers are used to diagnose diseases, categorize patients, and support treatment decisions. While proteins (6%–8%) are by far the second major component of plasma after water (90%–92%), metabolic, lipidomic, transcriptomic, and genomic readouts are also gaining traction as diagnostic tests in plasma. (3–6) Different omics readouts can be used in conjunction to improve diagnostic power. (7) Despite more than 20,000 diseases reported to affect humans (8), it is only for a small fraction of them that accurate, sensitive, and specific diagnostic tests exist.

The limited success of blood protein biomarkers is primarily due to analytical challenges that come with the proteomic analysis of blood plasma. On the one hand, the large biological variance between individuals and within individuals over time makes the discovery of reliable biomarker signatures difficult. Further, the steep dynamic range of human plasma, with an estimated dynamic range of 12–13 orders of magnitude, renders comprehensive proteome profiling challenging to any analytical technique. In the lower concentration range, thousands of proteins reside, mostly tissue leakage proteins and signaling molecules that could serve as biomarkers but are very challenging to measure, especially in an unbiased manner.[13]

9. Lung cancer in non-smokers: Scientists find how air pollution acts as a trigger

The World Health Organization (WHO) reports that lung cancer was the most common cause of cancer death in 2020, accounting for 1.8 million deaths globally. There are two main types of lung cancer, depending on the size of the cancer cells: small-cell lung cancer (SCLC) and non-small-cell lung cancer (NSCLC). NSCLC is a more common type, accounting for 8 out of 10 lung cancer diagnoses. It is a well-established fact that smoking increases the risk of lung cancer. Yet about 10%–20% of lung cancers happen in people who have never smoked or smoked fewer than 100 cigarettes in their lifetime, according to the Centers for Disease Control and Prevention (CDC).

When a team of researchers at the Francis Crick Institute (FCI) and University College London (UCL) started looking at never-smokers who developed non-small cell lung cancer, they noticed that most of them lived in areas where air pollution levels exceeded WHO guidelines. Although air pollution has been associated with lung cancer incidence for at least two decades, the exact mechanism by which small pollutant particles in the air cause lung cancer had not been identified.[14]

Researchers sought to understand the mechanism by which air pollution may induce non-small cell lung cancer in never-smokers. They found that fine particulate matter triggers inflammation in the lungs and causes lung cells with pre-existing mutations to start forming a tumor. The finding may pave the way for new potential approaches to lung cancer prevention and highlights the importance of reducing air pollution for human health.[15]

10. Strengthening the immune response to cancer

For patients with lymphoma, multiple myeloma, or certain types of leukemia, treatment with chimeric/imaginary antigen receptor T cells (CAR-T cells) is sometimes the last chance of overcoming cancer. The treatment involves taking T cells from the patient's blood and adding artificial receptors, the CARs, to them in the lab. As the guards of our immune system, T cells are on permanent patrol in our blood vessels and tissues, where they hunt down foreign structures. Equipped with CARs, T cells can also detect very specific surface structures on cancer cells. Once the CAR-T cells are returned to the patient by infusion, they circulate in the body as a kind of living drug that can bind to very specific tumor cells and destroy them. The engineered immune cells remain in the body permanently and multiply. If cancer flares up again, they'll go back into action. That's the theory, at least. But in practice, many patients still relapse. This is because the tumor cells can outwit the CAR-T cells by producing more of the protein EBAG9—and by causing the T cells to produce more of it, too. In T cells, EBAG9 inhibits the release of cytotoxic enzymes, which slows the desired immune response.

A month earlier, a team led by the last authors Dr. Armin Rehm and Dr. Uta Hoepken from the Max Delbrück Center for Molecular Medicine, Berlin, Germany, and the Helmholtz Association (MDC) showed in the journal *JCI Insight* that shutting down the EBAG9 gene in mice led to a sustained increase in the immune response to cancer. The mice also developed more T-memory cells. These cells are part of our immunological memory, which allows our immune system to respond better to a cancer antigen after encountering it previously.

Now the researchers have also shown these key findings in vitro, in human CAR-T cells. Writing in *Molecular Therapy*, the team says that this is the decisive step on the road to therapeutic use. "Shutting down EBAG9 allows the body to eradicate tumor cells earlier and more radically. As well as achieving longer-lasting therapeutic success, this could also create a real chance of cure," says Rehm.[16]

11. Releasing the brake for immunotherapy

As soon as the EBAG9 gene was discovered, researchers recognized that it played an important role in cancer. But it took a long time to identify what that role was. When the MDC team started working on it in 2009, they found that mice without the gene dealt with bacterial and viral infections much better than mice with the gene and that they formed more T- memory cells, which are of particular interest in tumor biology.

Then in 2015, lead author Dr. Anthea Wirges succeeded in curbing the synthesis of the EBAG9 protein using microRNA. For the latest study, she used microRNA to cultivate EBAG9-silenced CAR-T cells with different human leukemia or lymphoma cells. Just like in the mouse model, the silencing reduced tumor growth much more. Relapses also only developed much later.

"Releasing the EBAG9 brake allows the genetically engineered T cells to release more cytotoxic substances. However, they don't cause the strong cytokine storm that is typically a side effect of CAR therapy," says Wirges. In fact, the risk is minimized because fewer cells are used. "Switching off the immune brake works across the board. We can do it with every CAR-T cell that we produce, regardless of which type of blood cancer it targets." Clinical studies are the next step.

However, the first-in-line therapy for blood cancer will remain chemotherapy combined with conventional antibody therapy, as many patients respond very well to this. "CAR therapy only comes into play if the cancer returns. It's very expensive because it's an individual cellular product for a single person," says Hoepken, and a single treatment with such a product can save a life.

The EBAG9 work shows how important perseverance and patience are for researchers. Wirges was motivated by the prospect of her work having a real chance of clinical application. Rehm adds that "projects like this allow you to get to grips with a technique in basic research and then apply everything in translational research—right up to toxicological screening for the regulatory processes." Their project has now reached this last stage: The researchers will present their concept to the Paul Ehrlich Institute, Germany's biologics approval agency, in November. Thanks to their findings from animal models and the in vitro experiments using human cells, the team now knows that releasing the EBAG9 brake is highly effective and doesn't cause any more side effects than conventional CAR T therapy studies." Under the assumption that the research is progressing according to plan, the therapy "using EBAG9-silenced CAR-T cells could be available to patients in as little as two years' time."

12. Immunotherapy against cancer

For about 100 years, researchers have tried to target the body's own immune system to fight cancer cells. Two researchers, James Alison from the United States and Tasuku Honjo from Japan, in the 1990s, had a breakthrough that gave them the Nobel Prize in 2018, which has since been the foundation for immunotherapy for cancer. The two researchers started to investigate the mechanisms that allowed the cancer cells to avoid being caught by our immune system.

The first approval for the first checkpoint inhibitor against malignant melanoma already came in 2011. Since then, the checkpoint inhibitor method has been approved for several more malignant cancer types.[17]

My personal assessments of the most promising research projects are ongoing in 2022 and mentioned earlier.

There are so many new promising ideas and research directions being pursued today, and it is challenging to name the most promising ones. My choices are along several different directions:

- The new biopsy method is on the way to be able to image and analyze a sample tissue while still within the body. This will enable faster and much less invasive biopsies compared to the standard methodologies used up till now. My choice here is due to the great importance of being able to verify that the cells we are aiming at are the ones we really want to remove, which are cancer cells.
- The second one is the CAR-T treatments and potential improvements for the method.
- Finally, I am excited about the immunotherapy method with the checkpoint inhibitor being worked on even if the developments are at an early stage today.

Reference List, Chapter 17

1 www.cancer.gov/about-cancer/understanding/what-is-cancer
2 www.cancer.org/treatment/treatments-and-side-effects/treatment-types/immuno-therapy.html
3 Report from the American Cancer Society, 2018
4 www.cancer.net/navigating-cancer-care/prevention-and-healthy-living/understanding-cancer-risk
5 https://news.cancerresearchuk.org/2015/02/04/why-are-cancer-rates-increasing/
6 www.cdc.gov/cancer/lung/nonsmokers/index.htm
7 www.cancercenter.com/stage-one-cancer
8 www.cancer.gov/research/key-initiatives/moonshot-cancer-initiative/progress
9 https://medschool.duke.edu/news/developing-new-tools-fight-cancer
10 https://medium.com/geekculture/how-ai-and-x-rays-to-detect-explosives-could-also-identify-cancers-63dbd4c44fa3
11 https://jhoonline.biomedcentral.com/articles/10.1186/s13045-022-01392-3
12 www.cellsignal.com/pathways/angiogenesis-pathway
13 www.ncbi.nlm.nih.gov/pmc/articles/PMC9251764/
14 www.cdc.gov/cancer/lung/nonsmokers/index.htm
15 www.cancerresearchuk.org/about-cancer/what-is-cancer/body-systems-and-cancer/the-immune-system-and-cancer
16 https://ccr.cancer.gov/news/milestones-2019/article/releasing-the-brakes-on-the-immune-system
17 www.nhs.uk/conditions/stem-cell-transplant/

19

PRESENT STATUS OF CARDIOVASCULAR DISEASES IN THE YEAR 2022

19.1 Definition of Cardiovascular Disease

Cardiovascular disease (CVD) is a general term for conditions affecting the heart or blood vessels.

It's usually associated with a build-up of fatty deposits inside the arteries (arthrosclerosis) and an increased risk of blood clots.

It can also be associated with damage to arteries in organs such as the brain, heart, kidneys, and eyes.

CVD is one of the main causes of death and disability in the UK, but it can often largely be prevented by leading a healthy lifestyle.

The four main types are: coronary heart disease, stroke, peripheral arterial disease, aortic disease.[1]

The heart and the circulation of blood are really the motors in our body. The heart itself is a magnificent pump with advanced regulation. It serves all our organs with fresh blood during our lifetime, which means that it pumps our blood through an enormous number of beats during this time.

Let's say that we live to 80 years of age (we are getting older and older; it is a fact). This means that the heart beats 86,400 times every day (24 hours) if the number of beats per minute is 60. In one year, this means 31,536,000 beats. With a lifetime of 100 years, this means 3,153,600,000.

This is an amazing number of beats the heart must perform during a lifetime. This is far more than most mechanical equipment we are using today is capable of. If we live even longer, it is not surprising if there will be some wear on our heart-pumping capabilities, leading to heart complications in the future since we live longer and longer. If we add the many regulations of the blood system plus the blood vessels themselves, I am sure we all realize that the cardiovascular system is under a large amount of stress as we grow older.

19.2 Risk Factors for Getting a Cardiovascular Disease

- High blood pressure
- High low-density lipoprotein (LDL) cholesterol
- Diabetes
- Smoking and secondhand smoke exposure
- Obesity

DOI: 10.1201/9781003393320-23

- Unhealthy diet
- Physical inactivity

19.3 Incidence/Statistics for Cardiovascular Disease

- Each year, cardiovascular disease (CVD) causes 3.9 million deaths in Europe and over 1.8 million deaths in the European Union.
- CVD is the main cause of death in men in all but 12 countries of Europe and is the main cause of death in women in all but two countries.
- CVD by itself is the leading cause of mortality under 65 years in Europe.
- Overall, CVD is estimated to cost the European Union economy €210 billion a year.

19.4 Other Heart Diseases of Importance

19.4.1 Myocarditis

Myocarditis occurs when the heart muscle (myocardium) becomes inflamed. Inflammation occurs when your body's immune system responds to infections, for example. Myocarditis can be caused by viral infections or more systemic inflammatory conditions, such as autoimmune disorders. In severe cases of myocarditis, the heart muscle weakens and cannot pump blood effectively to other parts of your body.

19.4.2 Cardiomyopathy

Any disorder that affects the heart muscle is called cardiomyopathy. Cardiomyopathy causes the heart to lose its ability to pump blood well. In some cases, the heart rhythm also becomes disturbed. This leads to arrhythmias (irregular heartbeats). There are many causes of cardiomyopathy, including the following:

- Alcohol abuse
- High blood pressure
- Coronary artery disease
- Viral infections
- Certain medicines

Note: Many times, it is not possible to find the exact cause of the muscle disease.

19.5 Diagnostic Methods for Cardiovascular Disease

19.5.1 Noninvasive Tests

- Electrocardiogram (ECG): An ECG is a graphic measure of the electrical activity in your heart
- Stress EKG or echocardiogram
- Carotid ultrasound

- Abdominal ultrasound
- Holter monitor
- Cardiac catheterization and coronary angiography
- Electrophysiology study

19.5.2   Blood Tests for Heart Disease

19.5.2.1   Lipid Profile

The lipid profile includes the following:

- Total cholesterol
- LDL (low-density lipoprotein), the so-called bad cholesterol
- HDL (high-density lipoprotein), the so-called good cholesterol
- Triglycerides

19.5.3   Echocardiogram

An echocardiogram (echo) is an ultrasound of the heart. A small probe, like a microphone, called a transducer, is placed on the chest in various places. The ultrasound waves sent by the transducer bounce off the various parts of the heart. A computer in the machine determines the time it takes for the sound wave to return to the transducer and generates a picture with the data.

During the test, you will lie on your back or left side on a stretcher for about 45 minutes while the pictures are being recorded. The echocardiographer will review the pictures before sending you home to be sure all the necessary information has been obtained.

19.5.4   Stress ECG or Echocardiogram

Stress tests are performed to see how the heart performs under physical stress. The heart can be stressed with exercise on a treadmill or, in a few instances, a bicycle. If a person cannot exercise on a treadmill or bicycle, medications can be used to cause the heart rate to increase, simulating normal reactions of the heart to exercise.

During the stress test, you will wear EKG leads and wires while exercising so that the electrical signals of your heart can be recorded at the same time. Your blood pressure is monitored throughout the test. The stress test can be performed together with the echocardiogram, described earlier.

19.5.5   Nuclear Stress Test

Nuclear stress tests have two components to them: a treadmill (or chemical) stress test and a scan of the heart after injection of a radionuclide material. This material has been used safely for many years to determine the amount of blood the heart muscle is receiving during rest and stress. The scanning is done with a nuclear medicine (NM) camera.

19.5.6   Carotid Ultrasound

Carotid ultrasound is done to evaluate your risk of stroke. The sonographer presses the transducer gently against the sides of your neck, which sends images of your arteries to a computer screen for the technician to see. The technician monitors your blood flow through the carotid arteries on both sides of your neck to check for stenosis.

During the exam, you lie on your back on an examination table, and a small amount of warm gel is applied to your skin.

19.5.7   Abdominal Ultrasound

The doctor may also want you to have an abdominal ultrasound to screen for potential abdominal aortic aneurysm. The sonographer presses the transducer against the skin over your abdomen, moving from one area to another. The transducer sends images to a computer screen that the technician monitors. The technician monitors blood flow through your abdominal aorta to check for an aneurysm.

During the exam, you lie on your back on an examination table, and a small amount of warm gel is applied to your abdomen.

19.5.8   Holter Monitor

A Holter monitor is a small, portable machine that you wear for 24 to 48 hours. It enables continuous recording of your EKG as you go about your daily activities. You will be asked to keep a diary log of your activities and symptoms. This monitor can detect arrhythmias that might not show up on a resting EKG that only records for a few seconds.

19.5.9   Event Recorder

An event recorder (loop recorder) is a small, portable trans-telephonic monitor that may be worn for several weeks. This type of recorder is good for patients whose symptoms are infrequent.

The monitor loops a two- to five-minute recording into its memory, which is continually overwritten. When you experience symptoms, you press a record button on the monitor, which stores a correlating strip of EKG. The recordings are telephoned through to a 24-hour monitoring station and faxed directly to your doctor.

19.5.10   Invasive Tests

19.5.10.1   Cardiac Catheterization and Coronary Angiography

Cardiac catheterization is a common procedure that can help diagnose heart disease. In some cases, catheterization is also used to treat heart disease by opening blocked arteries with balloon angioplasty and stent placement.

Cardiac catheterization can show the following:

- If the blood vessels in your heart have narrowed.
- If your heart is pumping normally and blood is flowing correctly.
- If the valves in your heart are functioning normally.
- If you were born with any heart abnormalities.
- If the pressure in the heart and lungs is normal. If not, catheterization can help assess the problem.

During catheterization, the cardiologist inserts a long, flexible tube called a catheter into a blood vessel, either through the wrist artery or the groin artery, and gently guides it toward your heart under X-ray guidance. Once the catheter is in place, X-rays and other tests are done to help your doctor evaluate whether your coronary arteries are blocked and how well your heart is working.

At times, it might also be necessary to insert a small catheter into a vein to allow measurement of specific pressure in the heart and lungs. This procedure can be done either through a neck vein, arm vein, or groin vein.

19.5.10.2 Electrophysiology Study

An electrophysiology study (EP) is a recording of the electrical activity of the heart. This test helps your doctor determine the cause of your rhythm disturbance (arrhythmia) and the best treatment. During the test, the doctor may safely reproduce the arrhythmia and then give certain medications to see which one controls it best.

An EP study is performed in the Electrophysiology Laboratory, where you will lie on an X-ray table. As with cardiac catheterization, the doctor inserts a long, flexible tube—an electrode catheter—into a blood vessel, usually in the groin.

There are different stages in an EP study:

1. Recording the heart's electrical signals to assess electrical function.
2. Pacing the heart to bring on certain abnormal rhythms for observation under controlled conditions.
3. In some cases, performing an ablation procedure at the same time to destroy abnormal tissue, which may be causing the arrhythmia.

19.6 Therapeutic Methods for Cardiovascular Diseases

- Coronary angioplasty and stent implantation: Coronary angioplasty is a procedure that helps to improve blood flow to your heart
- Thrombolytic therapy
- Coronary artery bypass graft surgery (CABG)
- Artificial pacemaker surgery

- Defibrillation
- Heart valve surgery

19.7   Medicines

- Blood-thinning medicines
- Statins
- Beta-blockers
- Nitrates
- Angiotensin-converting enzyme (ACE) inhibitors
- Angiotensin-2 receptor blockers (ARBs)
- Calcium channel blockers
- Diuretics—reducing the water content in the body

19.8   Ongoing Interesting Research That Is Likely to or Can Materialize in Clinical Procedures in the Future

19.8.1   Stem Cell Treatment

In this technique, stem cells are injected into the heart with the expectation that they will evolve into cardiac cells and replace the damaged cells. This approach has enormous potential to help the heart heal itself, particularly when other treatment options are unavailable. Stem cell therapy continues to expand as short-term follow-up studies reveal blood vessel development, cellular regeneration, and improved perfusion in treated areas. Currently, clinical investigators are focusing on four conditions: acute myocardial infarction (MI), myocardial ischemia without revascularization, ischemic cardiomyopathy, and peripheral vascular disease. Researchers are considering the relative efficacies of different cell types and delivery methods for treating these conditions.

Owing to the ongoing controversy about the use of embryonic stem cells, alternative sources are being sought, including autologous cells from fat, bone marrow, skeletal muscle, or the heart itself. Animal models have recently shown that treatment is more effective if it relies on adult stem cells that express high levels of the aldehyde dehydrogenase enzyme. Stem cell delivery methods include trans endocardial injection into viable heart muscle or into the periphery of damaged myocardium, as well as catheter-based injection.[2]

19.8.2   Gene Therapy

In the developed world, coronary artery disease (CAD) is the leading cause of death and disability. The well-known risk factors for MI—increased age, tobacco use, obesity, lack of exercise, and hypertension—do not account for all cases of MI or CAD. Patients who have a premature MI often lack traditional risk factors. Researchers now know that genetic risk factors underlie many MIs. Genes affect high-density lipoprotein levels, programmed cell death, blood clotting, and in-stent restenosis.

Since 2001, the Texas Medical Center Genetics (TexGen) project[2] has been collecting genetic, clinical, and demographic data on the approximately 50,000 patients whom the participating institutions treat for cancer, cardiovascular disease, and stroke each year. By elucidating genetic risk factors, this information will help identify patients at increased risk for MIs, especially premature ones, leading to more efficient ways of predicting and preventing this complication.[3]

19.8.3   Noninvasive Diagnostic Imaging

Although coronary angiography has long been the gold standard for coronary artery assessment, emerging noninvasive technologies are improving the detection of CAD while posing less risk to patients. For example, 64-slice multidetector computerized tomography (CT)—a highly sensitive imaging technique—has become the preferred approach for diagnosing chest pain in low- or intermediate-risk patients who cannot undergo stress testing. By providing a coronary calcium score, the 64-slice system can also indicate the progress of coronary atherosclerosis or exclude CAD in emergency-room patients with equivocal acute chest pain.[4]

19.8.4   Cardiac Magnetic Resonance Imaging

Another emerging technology, cardiac magnetic resonance imaging (cardiac MRI), uses a multimodal approach to detect coronary artery stenosis without the need for radiation exposure. This approach first evaluates myocardial perfusion at rest and during stress. It then performs delayed-enhancement imaging to detect MI and necrosis. In CAD patients undergoing stem cell therapy, such imaging assesses the ventricular response to therapy and the status of myocardial perfusion. In addition, Cardiac MRI evaluates left ventricular function and detects scar tissue, providing a thorough assessment of the patient's cardiac health in less than one hour.[5]

19.8.5   Cardiovascular Surgery

Minimally invasive technologies are revolutionizing the field of cardiovascular surgery. The goal of minimally invasive surgery is to produce the positive outcomes typical of established procedures while lessening the trauma of surgical access. Although coronary artery bypasses and valve replacements will always be needed, the range of options for these procedures continues to expand.[6]

19.6.6   Minimal-Access Surgery

The degree of invasiveness of a cardiovascular surgical procedure depends on its incision size. Traditional access for cardiac procedures involves a full median sternotomy. However, with minimal-access surgery, numerous kinds of incisions present less invasive alternatives, such as partial sternotomies, limited-access thoracotomies without rib spreading, subxiphoid and subdiaphragmatic approaches, and catheter-based techniques. Many of these operations are performed with robotic techniques and video thoracoscopy. As far as possible, access is obtained through a natural body orifice or blood vessel.[7]

19.6.7   Laparoscopic (Keyhole) Surgery

Laparoscopy emerged in the 1980s for hernia repair*, appendectomy, and cholecystectomy. With time, it was extended to almost every internal organ, including the heart. Post-operatively, laparoscopy reduces pain, shortens recovery, and allows a quicker return to normal activities. Nevertheless, the technique involves a steep learning curve, and the operative time itself may be increased.

* A hernia occurs when an internal organ or other body part bulges out through the wall of muscle or tissue that normally contains it. Most hernias occur within the abdominal cavity, between the chest and the hips.[8]

19.6.8   Robot-Assisted Surgery

Robotic technology has been evolving as a minimally invasive means of treating cardiac ischemia and valve disease. The DaVinci™ Surgical System (Intuitive Surgical, Inc., Sunnyvale, CA) was approved by the US Food and Drug Administration (FDA) in 2002 for a wide variety of surgical procedures. It involves a surgeon sitting at a special console whose movements are mimicked by four robotic interactive arms. Vision is aided by a high-resolution 3D endoscope. The system enables surgeons to perform cardiac revascularization through a mini-thoracotomy without cardiopulmonary bypass or to perform a complex mitral valve repair. Moreover, by allowing a hybrid approach involving more than one surgical procedure (i.e., stent placement and aortic valve replacement), robot-assisted procedures lower morbidity and mortality, especially in high-risk patients with combined CAD and aortic valve disease.[9]

19.9   Obesity

Obesity has been said to be a ticking bomb due to being the reason for different serious cardiovascular diseases, like heart disease; diabetes; high blood pressure; and certain cancers.

> Half of world's population will be obese by 2035, the World Obesity Federation predicts.
>
> *BBC reported on March 2023*

> The findings show that overweight rates are rising fastest among kids, and that low to middle-income countries in Africa and Asia will undergo the starkest changes.[10]

People who seek medical treatment for obesity or an eating disorder do so with the hope their health plan will pay for part of it. But whether it's covered often comes down to a measure invented almost 200 years ago by a Belgian mathematician as part of his quest to use statistics to define the average man.

That work, done in the 1830s by Adolphe Quetelet, appealed to life insurance companies, which created ideal weight tables after the turn of the century. By the 1970s and 1980s, the measurement, now dubbed body mass index, was adopted to screen for and track obesity.

Now it's everywhere, using an equation—essentially a ratio of mass to height—to categorize patients as overweight, underweight, or at a healthy weight. It's appealingly simple, with a scale that designates adults who score between 18.5 and 24.9 as within a healthy range.

But critics, and they are widespread these days, say it was never meant as a health diagnostic tool. "BMI does not come from science or medicine," said Dr. Fatima Stanford, an obesity medicine specialist, and the equity director of the endocrine division at Massachusetts General Hospital.

She and other experts said BMI can be useful in tracking population-wide weight trends, but it falls short by failing to account for differences among ethnic groups, and it can target some people, including athletes, as overweight or obese because it does not distinguish between muscle mass and fat.

Still, BMI has become a standard tool to determine who is at most risk of getting health consequences of excess weight reasons and who qualifies for often, expensive treatments.

Despite the heavy debate surrounding BMI, the consensus is that people who are overweight or obese are at greater risk for a host of health problems, including diabetes, liver problems, osteoarthritis, high blood pressure, sleep apnea, and cardiovascular problems.

On the note of the heavily challenged BMI, it must be said that BMI works well when we are looking at a population or a large group of people but cannot say very much about the risk an individual is carrying. A person with a "good" BMI could still have a high risk of getting a cardiovascular event as the person's fat could be in the "wrong" place. However, a person who is overweight could still be without or have a low risk, as his fat could be in the "right" place.

Today, there are more modern available techniques that are much more exact and relevant measurements for obesity, and it includes the measurement of fat content. From these measurements, where an MRI is used, an individual body composition can be obtained.

The method is also capable of measuring fat content in a specific organ in the body; for instance, the liver. Scientists from the University in Linköping developed the technique, and today, it has been commercialized by AMRA AB (Figure 19.1). The method is used today within many scientific population studies and other research projects involving body fat.

Body Composition Profile – redefining obesity

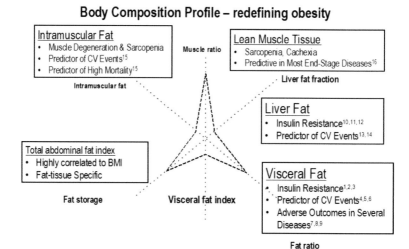

Figure 19.1   **An example of the results of AMRA AB's fat measurement with MRI.**
(Courtesy of AMRA Medical, Linköping, Sweden.)[11]

The breakthrough, making it a clinically used method for stratification and preventive medicine, still remains.

American researchers believe that they have identified a rare mutation that is protecting against abdominal obesity and metabolic syndrome. The ambition is that the discovery will lead to new treatments to reduce the risk of diabetes type 2 and cardiovascular diseases.

It is the pharmaceutical company Alnylam together with collaborators that found the mutation in the so-called INHBE gene and investigated its impact.

The development is built on data from sequencing more than 360,000 persons from the UK Biobank study and has been published in *Nature Communications*. The mutation by the INHBE gene that is expressed in the liver was found in every 587th person in the study. From the study, it was concluded that the INHBE gene contributed to a healthier distribution of body fat. The researchers also studied the monkeys. The overweight monkeys showed increased expression of the INHBE gene.

Alnylam Pharmaceuticals plan, via turning off the INHBE gene, to reduce the risk for abdominal fat issues, hereby avoiding the diseases following abdominal fat issues. The company wants to test the hypothesis to develop a pharmaceutical drug directed toward the INHBE gene.[12]

Reference List, Chapter 19

1 Ref. NIH, National Health Service
2 www.fda.gov/consumers/consumer-updates/how-gene-therapy-can-cure-or-treat-diseases

3 www.news-medical.net/health/What-is-the-Role-of-Non-invasive-Imaging-in-Diagnostics.aspx
4 https://my.clevelandclinic.org/health/diagnostics/21961-heart-mri
5 www.mayoclinic.org/departments-centers/cardiovascular-surgery/sections/overview/ovc-20123422
6 www.ncbi.nlm.nih.gov/pmc/articles/PMC1129081/
7 www.nhs.uk/conditions/laparoscopy/what-happens/
8 www.davincisurgery.com
9 https://amramedical.com/science/technology/
10 https://medicalxpress.com/news/2023-03-world-obese-health.html
11 www.ncbi.nlm.nih.gov/gene/83729
12 www.nature.com/articles/s41467-022-31757-8

20

PRESENT STATUS OF NEUROLOGICAL DISEASES IN THE YEAR 2022

20.1 Stroke

20.1.1 Definition

A stroke, sometimes called a brain attack, occurs when something blocks the blood supply to a part of the brain or when a blood vessel in the brain bursts. In either case, parts of the brain become damaged or die. A stroke can cause lasting brain damage, long-term disability, or even death.

A stroke occurs when blood circulation to the brain fails. Brain cells can die from decreased blood flow and the resulting lack of oxygen. There are two broad categories of stroke: those caused by a blockage of blood flow and those caused by bleeding into the brain. A blockage of a blood vessel in the brain or neck, called an ischemic stroke, is the most frequent cause of stroke and is responsible for about 80% of strokes. These blockages stem from three conditions: the formation of a clot within a blood vessel of the brain or neck, called thrombosis; the movement of a clot from another part of the body, such as the heart to the brain, called embolism; or a severe narrowing of an artery in or leading to the brain, called stenosis. Bleeding into the brain or the spaces surrounding the brain causes the second type of stroke, called a hemorrhagic stroke.

Two key steps you can take will lower your risk of death or disability from stroke: Control stroke's risk factors and know stroke's warning signs. Scientific research conducted by the NINDS (NIH National Institute of Neurological Disorders and Stroke) has identified warning signs and many risk factors.

20.1.2 Warning Signs

Warning signs are clues your body sends that your brain is not receiving enough oxygen. If you observe one or more of these signs of a stroke or brain attack, don't wait. Call emergency!

* Sudden numbness or weakness of the face, arm, or leg, especially on one side of the body
* Sudden confusion or trouble talking or understanding speech
* Sudden trouble seeing in one or both eyes
* Sudden trouble walking, dizziness, or loss of balance or coordination
* Sudden severe headache with no known cause

DOI: 10.1201/9781003393320-24

Other danger signs that may occur include double vision, drowsiness, and nausea or vomiting. Sometimes the warning signs may last only a few moments and then disappear. These brief episodes, known as transient ischemic attacks or TIAs, are sometimes called mini-strokes. Although brief, they identify an underlying serious condition that isn't going away without medical help. Unfortunately, since they clear up, many people ignore them. You should not! Paying attention to them can save your life.[1]

20.1.3   Risk Factors

A risk factor is a condition or behavior that occurs more frequently in those who have, or are at greater risk of getting, a disease than in those who don't. Having a risk factor for stroke doesn't mean you'll have a stroke. However, not having a risk factor doesn't mean you'll avoid a stroke. But your risk of stroke grows as the number and severity of risk factors increase.

20.1.3.1   Some Risk Factors for Stroke That Cannot Be Modified by Medical Treatment or Lifestyle Changes

Age: Stroke occurs in all age groups. Studies show the risk of stroke doubles for each decade between the ages of 55 and 85. But strokes can also occur in childhood or adolescence. Although stroke is often considered a disease of aging, the risk of stroke in childhood is highest during the perinatal period, which encompasses the last few months of fetal life and the first few weeks after birth.

Gender: Men have a higher risk for stroke in young and middle age, but rates even out at older ages, and more women die from stroke. Men generally do not live as long as women, so men are usually younger when they have their strokes and, therefore, have a higher rate of survival.

Ethnic groups/race: People from certain ethnic groups have a higher risk of stroke. For African Americans, stroke is more common and more deadly even in young and middle-aged adults than for any ethnic or other racial group in the United States. Studies show that the age-adjusted incidence of stroke is about twice as high in African Americans and Hispanic Americans as in Caucasians, and while stroke incidence has declined for whites since the 1990s, there has not been a decline for Hispanics or Black Americans. An important risk factor for African Americans is sickle cell disease, which can cause a narrowing of arteries and disrupt blood flow. The incidence of the various stroke subtypes also varies considerably in different ethnic groups.

Family history of stroke: Stroke seems to run in some families. Several factors may contribute to familial stroke. Members of a family might have a genetic tendency for stroke risk factors, such as an inherited predisposition for high blood pressure (hypertension) or diabetes. The influence of a common lifestyle among family members can also contribute to familial stroke.

20.1.3.2 Some of the Most Important Treatable Risk Factors for Stroke

20.1.3.2.1   High Blood Pressure or Hypertension

Hypertension is by far the most potent risk factor for stroke. Hypertension causes a two to four-fold increase in the risk of stroke before age 80. If your blood pressure is high, you and your doctor need to work out an individual strategy to bring it down to the normal range. Some ways that work: Maintain proper weight. Avoid drugs known to raise blood pressure. Eat right: Cut down on salt and eat fruits and vegetables to increase potassium in your diet. Exercise more. Your doctor may prescribe medicines that help lower blood pressure. Controlling blood pressure will also help you avoid heart disease, diabetes, and kidney failure.

20.1.3.2.2   Cigarette Smoking

Cigarette smoking causes about a two-fold increase in the risk of ischemic stroke and up to a four-fold increase in the risk of hemorrhagic stroke. It has been linked to the buildup of fatty substances (atherosclerosis) in the carotid artery, the main neck artery supplying blood to the brain. Blockage of this artery is the leading cause of stroke in Americans. Also, nicotine raises blood pressure; carbon monoxide from smoking reduces the amount of oxygen your blood can carry to the brain; and cigarette smoke makes your blood thicker and more likely to clot. Smoking also promotes aneurysm formation. Your doctor can recommend programs and medications that may help you quit smoking. By quitting, at any age, you also reduce your risk of lung disease, heart disease, and other cancers, including lung cancer.

20.1.3.2.3   Heart Disease

Common heart disorders, such as coronary artery disease, valve defects, irregular heartbeat (atrial fibrillation), and enlargement of one of the heart's chambers, can result in blood clots that may break loose and block vessels in or leading to the brain. Atrial fibrillation, which is more prevalent in older people, is responsible for one in four strokes after age 80 and is associated with higher mortality and disability. The most common blood vessel disease is atherosclerosis. Hypertension promotes atherosclerosis and causes mechanical damage to the walls of blood vessels. Your doctor will treat your heart disease and may also prescribe medication, such as aspirin, to help prevent the formation of clots. Your doctor may recommend surgery to clean out a clogged neck artery if you match a particular risk profile. If you are over 50, NINDS (National Institute of Neurological Disorders and Stroke) scientists believe you and your doctor should/could make a decision about aspirin therapy. A doctor can evaluate your risk factors and help you decide if you will benefit from aspirin or other blood-thinning therapy.[2]

20.1.3.2.4 Warning Signs or History of TIA or Stroke

If you experience a TIA, get help at once. If you've previously had a TIA or stroke, your risk of having a stroke is many times greater than someone who has never had one. Many communities encourage those with stroke warning signs to dial 911 for emergency medical assistance. If you have had a stroke in the past, it's important to reduce your risk of a second stroke. Your brain helps you recover from a stroke by asking the unaffected brain regions to do double duty. That means a second stroke can be twice as bad.[3]

20.1.3.2.5 Diabetes

We often think that diabetes affects only the body's ability to use sugar or glucose. But it also causes destructive changes in the blood vessels throughout the body, including the brain. Also, if blood glucose levels are high at the time of a stroke, then brain damage is usually more severe and extensive than when blood glucose is well-controlled. Hypertension is common among diabetics and accounts for much of their increased stroke risk. Treating diabetes can delay the onset of complications that increase the risk of stroke.[4]

20.1.3.2.6 Cholesterol Imbalance

Low-density lipoprotein cholesterol (LDL) carries cholesterol (a fatty substance) through the blood and delivers it to cells. Excess LDL can cause cholesterol to build up in blood vessels, leading to atherosclerosis. Atherosclerosis is the major cause of blood vessel narrowing, leading to both heart attack and stroke.[5]

20.1.3.2.7 Physical Inactivity and Obesity

Obesity and inactivity are associated with hypertension, diabetes, and heart disease. Waist circumference to hip circumference ratio equal to or above the mid-value for the population increases the risk of ischemic stroke three-fold.[6]

20.1.4 Alzheimer's Disease

20.1.4.1 Definition: Alzheimer's Disease

Alzheimer's disease (AD) is a neurodegenerative disease that usually starts slowly and progressively worsens (Figures 20.1 and 20.2). It is the cause of 60%–70% of cases of dementia. The most common early symptom is difficulty in remembering recent events. As the disease advances, symptoms can include problems with language, disorientation (including easily getting lost), mood swings, loss of motivation, self-neglect, and behavioral issues. As

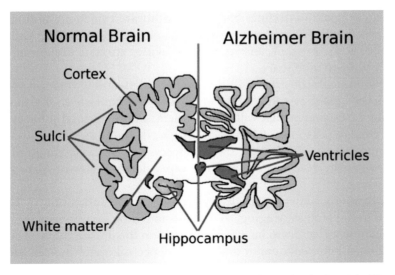

Figure 20.1   The difference between a healthy brain and a brain with AD. (en. wikiwand.com)[7]

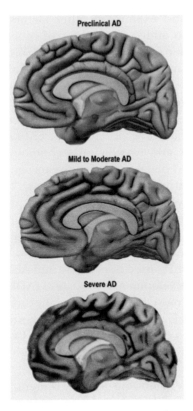

Figure 20.2   Different stages of Alzheimer's disease.[7]

a person's condition declines, they often withdraw from family and society. Gradually, bodily functions are lost, ultimately leading to death. Although the speed of progression can vary, the typical life expectancy following diagnosis is three to nine years.

A combination of drugs will be needed to effectively treat or prevent Alzheimer's disease, and leading experts say we have entered a new era of drug development that will deliver them. In an editorial published in the *Journal of Prevention of Alzheimer's Disease*, the authors say the two most important factors driving us toward success are the wide range of new drug targets in development and the rapid development of Alzheimer's biomarkers.

"Alzheimer's is a complex disease caused by a combination of factors related to the biology of aging, so it stands to reason we will need to treat a combination of factors to have a real impact on the disease," says co-author Dr. Howard Fillit, co-founder and chief science officer of the Alzheimer's Drug Discovery Foundation (ADDF).

There are currently 143 drugs in development to fight Alzheimer's, including 119 designed to slow or stop the disease. While amyloid-busting drugs dominated research not long ago, today, there are more Alzheimer's drug trials targeting and examining other factors than these proteins. Ongoing trials are also addressing a host of other age-related changes implicated in Alzheimer's, including in metabolism, vascular function, epigenetics (changes in gene regulation without alterations in the DNA sequence), and nerve cell formation.

Equally important are significant advancements in biomarkers, which are necessary for early diagnosis and selective recruitment of the right patients for the right clinical trials. The development of biomarkers—in the form of blood tests, eye scans, and even digital, technology-based tests—can help with early detection and diagnosis. Just 10 years ago, the only way to diagnose Alzheimer's was through postmortem autopsy. Today, brain PET scans, spinal fluid tests, and even a simple blood test can provide insights into the condition of the Alzheimer's brain.

"Biomarkers ensure the right patients are enrolled in each clinical trial and give researchers the means to evaluate their response to treatment," says co-author Yuko Hara, PhD, director of Aging and Alzheimer's Prevention at the Alzheimer's Drug Development Foundation (ADDF). "Biomarkers make clinical trials more and more rigorous, especially early-stage trials where it is vital to determine quickly whether treatment shows promise so that clinical trial dollars are spent on treatments that are most likely to work."

The ADDF organization is supported by Jeff Bezos and Bill Gates, among many others.

The ADDF gave the following announcement, November 29, 2022: "Today's results show that *lecanemab* slows cognitive decline, which is welcome news for the millions of patients and families living with Alzheimer's," said Dr. Howard Fillit, co-founder and chief science officer at the ADDF. "But this is only a start to stopping Alzheimer's in its tracks. We have a lot of ground to cover to get from the 27% slowing *Lecanemab* offers to our goal of slowing cognitive decline by 100%.

As a neuroscientist and geriatrician, I am more optimistic than ever about our ability to prevent, diagnose and treat Alzheimer's disease. . . . With an increasing ability to diagnose individual causes of Alzheimer's in each patient, and well over 100 different drugs in the research pipeline, we are closer than ever to offering patients a personalized combination approach to their disease, just as we do for cancer and cardiovascular disease."[8]

Note: Some interesting videos from the National Institutes of Health (NIH) in the United States can be viewed via the address referenced later.[9]

20.1.5   Risk Factors

The biggest risk factor for Alzheimer's and other forms of dementia is older age, which people obviously cannot change. Genetic susceptibility is another major player; people who carry a gene variant called APOE4, for example, have a higher likelihood of developing Alzheimer's than non-carriers do.

Certain genes can increase the risk of developing dementia, including Alzheimer's disease.

One of the most significant genetic risk factors is a form of the apolipoprotein E gene called APOE4.

About 25% of people carry one copy of APOE4, and 2% to 3% carry two copies. APOE4 is the strongest risk factor gene for Alzheimer's disease, although inheriting APOE4 does not mean a person will develop the disease.

More than 55 million people worldwide are believed to be living with dementia, according to the World Health Organization. And women are likely to be twice as affected by dementia as men.

Dementia is an umbrella term for a group of symptoms affecting memory, thinking, and social abilities. It's not one disease. And Alzheimer's disease is the most common form of dementia.

Dr. Ronald Petersen, director of the Alzheimer's Disease Research Center at Mayo Clinic, says you can't prevent dementia, but you can reduce some of your dementia risks. In fact, there are a dozen risk factors that are possible to avoid or at least possible to minimize.[10]

20.2   Ongoing Interesting Research That Is Likely to or Can Materialize in Clinical Procedures in the Future

The most focus and research today is on the neuro degenerative diseases of the brain. In addition to Alzheimer's disease, it is Parkinson's disease, Huntingdon's disease, amyotrophic lateral sclerosis (ALS), multiple sclerosis, and migraine.

There are certainly more diseases in the brain, but the previously mentioned ones are the most common, and this is why my focus is on those mentioned.

1. New biomarker could help diagnose Alzheimer's disease early
by American Chemical Society

A definitive diagnosis of Alzheimer's disease (AD) was once only possible after someone had died, but recent biomarker studies have led to the development of imaging and spinal fluid tests for those still living. However, the tests can only monitor severe disease, differentiating advanced AD from related disorders. Reporting in *ACS Chemical Neuroscience*, researchers have now identified a biomarker that could help physicians diagnose AD earlier, as a patient transitions into mild cognitive impairment (MCI).

When hunting for AD biomarkers, some researchers have turned to the study of subtle changes in a protein called tau. These changes, or posttranslational modifications, can make the tau protein more likely to clump, which leads to neuron loss and impaired memory. Two such modifications involve the phosphorylation of tau at specific amino acids, resulting in versions called p-tau181 and p-tau217. These biomarkers have been shown to effectively differentiate AD tissues from those of people with other neurodegenerative diseases.

Because it's helpful to have many biomarkers in the physicians' toolbox, Bin Xu, Jerry Wang, Ling Wu, and colleagues sought additional p-tau biomarkers that could be effective AD diagnostics, or that could perhaps catch AD at its early stages.[11]

2. Detecting Alzheimer's disease in the blood
by Hokkaido University

Researchers from Hokkaido University and Toppan have developed a method to detect the buildup of amyloid β in the brain, a characteristic of Alzheimer's disease, from biomarkers in blood samples.

A team of scientists from Hokkaido University and Toppan, led by Specially Appointed Associate Professor Kohei Yuyama at the Faculty of Advanced Life Science, Hokkaido University, have developed a biosensing technology that can detect Aβ-binding exosomes in the blood of mice, which increase as Aβ accumulates in the brain. Their research was published in the journal *Alzheimer's Research & Therapy*.

Clinical trials of the technology are currently underway in humans. This highly sensitive idICA technology is the first application of ICA that enables highly sensitive detection of exosomes that retain specific surface molecules from a small amount of blood without the need to learn special techniques; as it is applicable to exosome biomarkers in general, it can also be adapted for use in the diagnosis of other diseases.[12]

3. Biomarkers for Parkinson's disease sought through imaging
by Beth Miller, Washington University School of Medicine in St. Louis

More than 10 million people worldwide live with Parkinson's disease, a progressive neurodegenerative disorder that affects movement, balance, and thinking. The severity of the disease is measured through external symptoms, as there are no effective biomarkers that indicate the phase of the illness.

A team of engineers, physicians, and researchers at Washington University in St. Louis, led by Abhinav K. Jha in the McKelvey School of Engineering, has collaborated to create an imaging method that allows them to get an accurate measurement of the dopamine transporter, a protein important in movement, in three regions in the brain associated with Parkinson's disease. The results of their research appeared in *Medical Physics*, published in August 2022.

The team developed a way to calculate the uptake of dopamine transporter using single-photon emission computerized tomography (SPECT) in the caudate, putamen, and globus pallidus regions in the brain in simulation studies.

While most studies on developing biomarkers for Parkinson's disease have focused on measuring the dopamine transporter uptake within caudate and putamen, such measures may only correlate with severity in early Parkinson's disease. That leaves an important need for biomarkers that can measure the severity throughout the range of the disease. To reach this goal, Perlmutter, a prominent physician and researcher in Parkinson's disease, encouraged Jha to determine if the dopamine transporter uptake within the globus pallidus could serve as a biomarker.

"This project leads the way to developing new measures of Parkinson disease severity," Perlmutter said. "Such measures are critically important to development of new treatments to slow disease progression."[13]

4. Bioartic AB, a Swedish biomedicine research company, receives an American patent for transport method to pass the blood–brain barrier for drugs

Bioartic is using its technology platform for the development of treatments for Alzheimer's disease, Parkinson's disease, and other diseases in the central nervous system.

The blood–brain barrier protects the brain from foreign substances entering the brain. This also includes drugs. This development will help many researchers to make a way into the brain for new drug aspirants.[14]

5. New Alzheimer's drug shows promise in phase 3 clinical trial

The study, conducted at sites in Japan, China, Europe, and the United States, included 1,795 participants with mild cognitive impairment due to Alzheimer's disease (AD). The presence of amyloid plaques was confirmed in all participants.

The findings from a phase 3 clinical trial have yet to be peer-reviewed in any medical journal. But according to a company news release, "lecanemab treatment met the primary endpoint and reduced clinical decline on the global cognitive and functional scale, CDR-SB, compared with placebo at 18 months, by 27%."

Lecanemab is a monoclonal antibody that binds to neutralize and eliminate the amyloid-beta aggregates in the brain.

I think it is a fantastic achievement, as this is the first drug that has had any positive effect against Alzheimer's disease. It is also linked to a method where the drug has passed the blood–brain barrier. The researchers are not there yet, but a small step has been taken toward a drug for reducing the clinical decline in Alzheimer's disease and is, therefore, encouraging.

6. **Human Brain Project researchers identify new marker of ALS outcome**
   by Roberto Inchingolo, Human Brain Project

A study by Human Brain Project (HBP) researchers has identified a new marker for predicting the clinical outcome of patients with amyotrophic lateral sclerosis (ALS) through magnetoencephalography. This marker can be measured in the brain during its resting state and highlights the importance of brain flexibility for ALS patients. The study has been led by the Institute de Neurosciences des System in Marseille, in collaboration with Consiglio Nazionale delle Ricerche, Parthenope University of Naples, and Institute of Diagnosis and Care Hermitage Capodimonte in Naples, and the Monash University in Melbourne. It was published online on September 30, 2022, in *Neurology*.

ALS is a neurodegenerative disease of the brain and spinal cord that causes loss of muscle control. The ability to move, speaking, and eventually, breathe is progressively impaired. There is no known cure, but treatments to improve symptoms, including magnetic stimulation, are being tested.[15]

7. **Ultra-high-res MRI reveals migraine brain changes**

   Meeting Announcement
   News Release: November 23, 2022
   Radiological Society of North America

Migraine is a common, often debilitating condition, involving a severe recurring headache. Migraines may also cause nausea, weakness, and light sensitivity. According to the American Migraine Foundation, over 37 million people in the United States are affected by migraine, and up to 148 million people worldwide suffer from chronic migraine.

Perivascular spaces are fluid-filled spaces surrounding blood vessels in the brain. They are often located in the basal ganglia and white matter of the cerebrum and along the optic tract. Perivascular spaces are affected by several factors, including abnormalities in the blood–brain barrier and inflammation. Enlarged perivascular spaces can be a signal of underlying small vessel disease "in people with chronic migraine and episodic migraine without aura, there are significant changes in the perivascular spaces of a brain region called the centrum 'semiovale'," said study co-author Wilson Xu, an MD candidate at Keck School of Medicine of the University of Southern California in Los Angeles. "These changes have never been reported before."

Xu and colleagues set out to determine the association between migraine and enlarged perivascular spaces. The researchers used ultra-high-field 7T MRI to compare structural microvascular changes in different types of migraine.[16]

8.   Stroke: Researchers develop AI model to predict a person's 10-year risk

Recently, researchers from Massachusetts General Hospital developed a deep learning model using artificial intelligence (AI) and a single chest X-ray to help predict a person's 10-year risk of dying from a stroke or heart attack.

Using a chest X-ray to predict heart disease: According to Dr. Nicole Weinberg, a cardiologist at Providence Saint John's Health Center in Santa Monica, California, who is not involved in the new study, many people may assume that a chest X-ray only looks at the lungs.

But when a radiologist takes a picture of a person's chest, they will also see other organs in the area of the lungs, including the heart.

The team used a CXR-CVD system that was trained to search more than 147,000 chest X-ray images from almost 41,000 participants in a cancer screening trial and spot patterns associated with cardiovascular disease. Once developed, the system could predict a person's 10-year risk of having a stroke or heart attack from a single chest X-ray.

"Identifying people with higher risk for cardiovascular disease early is important, and more tools to help identify those at risk is always useful," Dr. Wong told MNT:

> This study did a great job of correlating with the current tool that cardiologists use, the ASCVD risk score, but to see based on where they risk-stratify somebody what happens to that person's risk of heart attack and stroke 10 or 20 years down the road with just chest X-ray as the tool might be helpful.[17]

9.   Alzheimer's disease: Urine biomarker may provide early detection.
Researchers from Shanghai Jiao Tong University and WuXi Diagnostics Innovation Research Institute in China collaborated to analyze the role of formic acid as an Alzheimer's disease urinary biomarker

In a recent study, researchers in China recruited hundreds of participants with healthy cognition or dementia to study biomarkers for Alzheimer's disease that can be detected early. The researchers focused their study on urinary formic acid, a formaldehyde product. By checking participants' formic acid levels, the researchers learned that higher levels found in urine may point to impaired cognition. The scientists hope the findings will lead to testing for early detection of Alzheimer's that is inexpensive and accessible.

After comparing the formic acid levels among each group, the researchers learned that there was a difference among the participants with healthy cognition versus those with at least some degree of impairment.

If further studies indicate that urinary formic acid can detect cognitive decline, it may prove to be an accessible, affordable test.

My personal assessments of the most promising research projects that are ongoing in 2022 and mentioned earlier.

My personal favorites of the eight projects described earlier are the following three:

- The project with the first drug against Alzheimer's disease, obtaining positive results in a phase 3 study, I see as a breakthrough that could lead to new drugs. It is also linked to a new development being able to pass through the blood–brain barrier. This fact can help other scientists, with the aim to get into the brain with other pharmaceuticals.
- Today, we know how to diagnose AD, with primarily PET and, if at a later stage also, with MRI. These two modalities are rather overloaded with patients, and hence, a blood test method would be preferred for the diagnosis of AD.
- I am also very positive about the project in migraine detection (number 7) with 7T MRI. It is a very recent project, but I hope that this can develop into a practical solution that can lead to a diagnostic tool and eventually also to treatment. The use of a 7T unit is not for everyone, but most likely, it will also become available in lower field strengths.

Reference List, Chapter 20

1 www.mayoclinic.org/diseases-conditions/stroke/symptoms-causes/syc-20350113
2 www.heartandstroke.ca/stroke/risk-and-prevention/risk-factors-you-cannot-change
3 www.mayoclinic.org/diseases-conditions/transient-ischemic-attack/symptoms-causes/syc-20355679
4 www.diabetes.org.uk/guide-to-diabetes/complications/stroke
5 www.stroke.org.uk/what-is-stroke/are-you-at-risk-of-stroke/high-cholesterol
6 www.ncbi.nlm.nih.gov/pmc/articles/PMC6117021/
7 https://commons.wikimedia.org/w/index.php?search=alzheimers+disease&title=Special:MediaSearch&go=Go&type=image360) www.alzdiscovery.org
8 www.youtube.com/watch?v=ezpi8J1UQA0
9 www.cdc.gov/aging/publications/features/reducing-risk-of-alzheimers-disease/index.htm
10 www.sciencedaily.com/releases/2022/11/221109085756.htm

11 www.global.hokudai.ac.jp/blog/detecting-alzheimers-disease-in-the-blood/
12 https://engineering.wustl.edu/news/2022/Biomarkers-for-Parkinsons-disease-sought-through-imaging.html
13 www.nejm.org/doi/full/10.1056/NEJMoa2212948
14 www.humanbrainproject.eu/en/follow-hbp/news/2022/10/03/human-brain-project-researchers-identify-new-marker-als-outcome/
15 www.eurekalert.org/news-releases/971466
16 www.medicalnewstoday.com/articles/stroke-researchers-use-ai-model-to-predict-10-year-risk-heart-disease
17 www.medicalnewstoday.com/articles/alzheimers-disease-urine-biomarker-shown-to-provide-early-detection

21

ARTIFICIAL INTELLIGENCE

It is almost impossible to read or write today anything in science without touching on artificial intelligence in some shape. This book is no difference in this respect. Moreover, in the field of medical and technology science, AI is used in many areas and disciplines. Let's look at what and where AI is used in technology and medical science.

21.1 Definition

Artificial intelligence: A feature where machines/computers learn to perform tasks, rather than simply carry out computations that are input by human users.

21.2 Different Types of AI Used in Medicine

Machine learning: An approach to AI in which a computer algorithm (a set of rules and procedures) is developed to analyze and make predictions from data that is fed into the system.

Neural networks: A machine learning approach modeled after the brain in which algorithms process signals via interconnected nodes called artificial neurons.

Mimicking biological nervous systems: Artificial neural networks have been used successfully to recognize and predict patterns of neural signals involved in brain function.

21.3 AI Is Being Used to Improve Medical Care and Biomedical Research

Radiology: The ability of AI to interpret imaging results may aid in detecting a very small change in an image that a clinician might miss. Moreover, the AI can help by giving the radiologist a heads-up in a situation complicated to interpret. A good example is the reading of a mammography image in a screening program.

Imaging: One example is the use of AI to evaluate how an individual will look after facial and cleft palate surgery.

Telehealth: Wearable devices allow for constant monitoring of a patient and detecting physiological changes that may provide early warning signs of an event such as an asthma attack or atrial fibrillation.

DOI: 10.1201/9781003393320-25

Clinical care: A large focus of AI in the healthcare sector is in clinical decision support systems, which use health observations and case knowledge to assist with treatment decisions.

Drug development: In drug development, AI is being used in several ways. In one application, AI can help in the early phase when a large number of potential molecules/compounds are being considered before entering phase 3. Here, AI can be of great help to avoid having too many candidates in this very expensive step in drug development.[1]

My personal view: I think there is great potential to introduce and use AI in many types of medical research. My worry at the moment is that AI is in the middle of a big hype, and by moving too fast into many new application areas, it can create many types of setbacks.

In order to work properly, there needs to be a large database, and this point is easy to forget.

The experience I have is from the days when we introduced mammography in Sweden in the mid-1980s. The radiologists that read all the films (we used silver-based films those days) became tired or got disturbed with an increased risk of missing small cancers. We then built a prototype system where we had a high-resolution TV camera to look at each film overnight (we did not have digital reading systems in those days). The following day, we had the radiologist look at the cases where our AI system saw something that was suspicious. Our very simple AI system found now and then suspicious areas of the images, but most of the time, other parameters had an impact on the discoveries from the AI system, like exposure conditions and other small issues that the radiologist filtered out very easily. The advantage of the system was that it gave the radiologists a sort of safety net in case they got tired or was distracted by the environment of the reading. The key thing was that it was always the radiologist that took the decisions.

My concern is that as soon as we believe too much in the reading capability of a programmed computer, the risks for mistakes increase and systematic errors can become an issue for any outcome.

Reference List, Chapter 21

1 www.mckinsey.com/industries/life-sciences/our-insights/how-ai-could-revolutionize-drug-discovery

22

GENOMICS

The human genome is made up of about 3.1 billion DNA subunits, pairs of chemical bases known by the letters A, C, G, and T (A, adenine; C, cytosine; G, guanine; and T, thymine).

Genes are strings of these lettered pairs that contain instructions for making proteins, the building blocks of life. Humans have about 30,000 genes, organized in 23 groups called chromosomes that are found in the nucleus of every cell in our body.

In 2021, after two decades of work on the human reference genome, the first truly complete sequence of the human genome was finished.

This work adds new genetic information to the human genome, corrects previous errors, and reveals long stretches of DNA known to play important roles in both evolution and disease. A version of the research was published last year before being reviewed by scientific peers.[1]

Every other organism on Earth contains the molecular instructions for life, called deoxyribonucleic acid or DNA. Encoded within this DNA are the directions for traits as diverse as the color of a person's eyes, the scent of a rose, and the way in which bacteria infect a lung cell.

Recently, the Nobel Prize in Medicine for 2022 was given to Swedish scientist Svante Pääbo, working at the Max Plank Institute in Leipzig. The Nobel Prize in Physiology or Medicine this year, 2022, will be given for a very unusual discovery, but it has an impact on our DNA for some of us even today.

New, interesting work has been presented that shows our genomic relations with the Neanderthals that lived between 500,000 and 40,000 years earlier. This can have a significant impact on the effect of the drugs we consume today. The drugs can give either a stronger or a less strong effect, depending on the individual person's genome in relation to the Neanderthal genome.

Earlier discoveries that were made public in 2022 was the first sequenced genome from an individual who lived in Pompeii, Italy, and died in connection with the eruption of Mount Vesuvius, in 79 CE.[2]

The sequencing of the human genome has continuously become faster and faster but also cheaper and cheaper.

DOI: 10.1201/9781003393320-26

Let's update ourselves on the Human Genome Project:

- The Human Genome Project was initiated in 1990 and was finished in 2003 and cost billions of dollars. The funding came from the American government, through the NIH (National Institutes of Health), and from many different institutions around the world. In 2003, 85% of the human genome was done.
- The level of complete genome was achieved in May 2021. There was still 0.3% left to be totally complete, and this was finished in January 2022.
- The sequencing technique has been developed, and today, it takes 6–8 weeks to receive the information, and it costs US$300–600.
- There are different possible tests you can order, and most tests can be done at your home (saliva or blood are the most common test). The sample is then sent to the sequencing and analysis company.[3]
- Newly emerging NGS (next-generation sequencing) technologies and instruments have further contributed to a significant decrease in the cost of sequencing nearing the mark of $1,000 per genome sequencing.

Many new initiatives will be dependent on the genetic profiling capability we can offer today. The trend of personalized medicine, with diagnosis and treatment being adapted to a specific person and not a treatment that is one-size-fits-all like we are doing today. We need many changes in order to reach an individualized approach to healthcare, while everybody aims for reaching this goal.[4]

Reference List, Chapter 22

1 www.genome.gov/about-genomics/educational-resources/fact-sheets/human-genome-project
2 www.nobelprize.org/prizes/medicine/2022/paabo/facts/
3 www.ncbi.nlm.nih.gov/pmc/articles/PMC3841808/
4 www.illumina.com/science/technology/next-generation-sequencing.html

23

WHAT ABOUT HEALTHCARE IN THE DEVELOPING WORLD?

Today, approximately half of the world's population does not have access to what we in the Western world call healthcare.

This is, unfortunately, the fact and has been reported by many organizations and researchers and specifically the WHO, the World Health Organization.

It is somewhat difficult for us living in the Western world to understand. This stark fact presents a troubling counterpoint to the satisfaction we take from the remarkable advances in medicine and medical technology—the innovative new treatments being developed and the effective cures that were unimaginable some decades ago.

The challenge facing everyone who truly cares about the future of healthcare is finding ways to bring care to all those who need it, when they need it, wherever they may be.

This statement/goal is not easy to live up to in most of the developing world. This includes most parts of Africa and many parts of Asia.

In Europe, we also have countries or areas in countries where the healthcare level suffers from coverage and a fair level of healthcare for the population.

In fact, we are also struggling in areas in Sweden due to long distances and not enough coverage of hospitals and clinics, specifically in the rural areas in the far north. Even where we have hospitals, it is challenging to staff these hospital and clinics with the requisite competence.

When I say "struggling," I mean that we are still on a level where solutions and quick fixes can be found, so we are struggling on a different level than how poor countries are.

Africa bears "more than 24% of the global burden of disease, but has access to only 3% of health workers and less than 1% of the world's financial resources," according to WHO. The poor status of health systems in many African countries is disturbing facts. These facts are not open to quick fixes, and it will take many years to build stable reasonable healthcare for many countries in Africa.

Another challenge for these countries is the number of medical professionals and their competence. Even if the Western world is also seeing recruitment issues, it is another dimension in Africa and parts of Asia.

There is some good news as well. Everywhere, at least, it is widespread—the density of mobile phones is high. When the Western world started to

DOI: 10.1201/9781003393320-27

build our healthcare systems, we built our clinics and hospitals with the aim of physical contact only, as we did not have mobile technology. Today, we are trying to integrate mobile technology into our health infrastructures, which goes rather slowly. Digital healthcare methods can hopefully speed up the development of an efficient digitized healthcare system where hospitals and clinics are used only for the patients that really need specialist care. Primary care could be very much more effective if we used the digital tool much more than physical appointments. This is a possible and potential method we have learned during the Covid-19 pandemic we are having worldwide today. There is a huge potential in the many techniques and applications where our mobile phones can be used instead of a physical visit to a doctor. The technique is already available and ready to be used in order to evaluate and refine it further.

Maybe the developing world doesn't have to do all the mistakes the developed world has done. Especially when it comes to investing in healthcare technology that serves a very small part of the population while the real advantage could be to invest more in technology that serves and helps a large group of the population.

I read an article that was from 2008 where WHO, the World Health Organization, looked at the health situation in Africa. The conclusion was very negative and shocking to me. There were a lot of things missing within the health system in most African countries, like qualified doctors, nurses, and medicines, although Africa had a dominating position when it comes to diseases. What struck me the most was the conclusion from WHO. Here's a quote from this article:

> Effective, public health interventions are available to curb the heavy disease burden in Africa. Unfortunately, health systems are too weak to deliver those interventions efficiently and equitably to people who need them, when and where needed.
>
> Fortunately, the health policy-makers know what actions ought to be implemented to strengthen health systems. However, it might not be possible to adequately implement those **actions without a concerted and coordinated fight against corruption**, sustained domestic and external investment in social sectors (i.e., health, education, water, sanitation), and enabling macroeconomic and political (i.e., internally secure) environment.[1]

My immediate thought was to find more recent documentation on the progress made. Yes, I found some, and there has been progress between 2008 and 2017.

Some of the progress that has been made includes:

- Gains made in fighting against malaria
- It's time to rethink medical insurance

- Diagnosing Africa's medical brain drain
- Lifestyle diseases pose a new burden for Africa
- Public health schemes: Getting it right
- Dr. Matshidiso Moeti: We can improve health systems in Africa
- Mental illness: Invisible but devastating
- India's medical tourism gets Africans' attention
- Taking health services to remote areas
- Dying from lack of medicines

Looking at the preceding titles, it could almost be any of our countries in Europe, America, Asia, or Australia.

Another good thing is that corruption is not mentioned in this latest WHO report.[2]

Reference List, Chapter 23

1 www.afro.who.int/sites/default/files/sessions/documents/State%20of%20 health%20in%20the%20 African%20Region.pdf
2 www.afro.who.int/sites/default/files/2018-08/English%20-%20Illustrative%20 report%20%26%20Summary%20Report%202017-2018.pdf

24

WHAT TYPE OF HEALTHCARE CAN WE EXPECT IN THE FUTURE?

It is always exciting to try and look into the future. Or maybe it is not so interesting?

Albert Einstein said, "I never think about the future, it comes soon enough!"

Still, I think it is somewhat interesting and valuable to look at what we have today and see/think about where the new ideas and thoughts could lead in the future.

I would like to suggest a few areas where new and important changes will happen in the (near) future.

24.1 Imaging

It is sometimes said that 1 image says more than 10 words. All our traditional modalities will continue to deliver improved techniques and, hereby, increase the value of imaging. The growing modality seen from an expanding applications point of view is MRI. The modality is expanding in several directions:

1. A new technique enabling almost zero helium consumption so low that no quench tube is needed. This will dramatically reduce both installation costs as well as running costs.
2. The modality is expanding also into lower field strengths, enabling MRI to be taken to the patient and again expanding with new applications.
3. The rather new modality of PET/MRI is starting to give very exciting results with the morphological one as the base and then the functional one overlaid. This makes the combined modality of PET/MRI to be more specific.

The next modality that is under huge and important development is computerized tomography (CT):

1. CT has developed into a modality that is used in most situations in a hospital. In the intensive care units, CT is the prime modality and will remain so also in the foreseeable time.
2. CTs have up till now been using an energy integration technique when the X-ray photons have passed the patients and reached the detector. A few years back, a new detector technology has been developed. It is

DOI: 10.1201/9781003393320-28

called photon-counting CT (PCCT). With this technique, the signal in each detector element is depending on how many photons are counted. The detector element is giving us the spatial position. In a photon-counting detector, we are also able to measure the energy by having the incoming photons collected in different energy bins. The energy of the photons passing the patient is important, as it gives us more information than if you only integrate the signal from all the incoming photons in every single moment. The new technique Is giving higher spatial resolution and reduced radiation dose. The radiation dose is an important parameter, as it is CT that is giving the dominating contribution to the radiation population dose of all medications used radiation. All vendors will have PCCT on their product line within the next few years.

3. Positron-emission tomography (PET) and single-photon emission computerized tomography (SPECT) will become increasingly important when not only the morphological image is considered but merely the function of organs and tissues. The view I have is that these modalities, depending on easy access to radiopharmaceuticals, could flourish as soon as we have a fully automated and simplified process of the radiotracers close to the scanners. This is a must if we want to use endogenous (tracers that are naturally available in our bodies, like oxygen, nitrogen, and carbon). These substances all have short half-lives to be transported. It is well documented that the world's clinicians are at a breaking point due to an overload of work. Nearly half of all critical care physicians, neurologists, and cardiologists say that they are burned out, along with over one in four radiologists. It's a long-standing issue that clinical staff experienced burnout before, under, and after the Covid-19 pandemic. After the very intense pandemic crises, the situation of overloaded and pressured clinicians has been on the agenda in many countries. Several people have raised voices that AI could help on this topic.

24.2   The Digitization Era Continues

New possibilities in healthcare enabled by digital health and artificial intelligence will enable new developments and more automatic technologies and processes.

24.3   Telemedicine Will Be Integrated into Healthcare Delivery

The Covid-19 pandemic led to wider adoption of telemedicine worldwide, transforming this once underutilized form of care delivery from obscure to ubiquitous almost overnight. Hospitals will continue to adopt this reliable and cost-effective technology to deliver care as a matter of urgency in 2022.

24.4   Use of Healthcare Resources in a More Effective Manner Is Critical from Cost and Resource Use

The faster we can get the expertise in connection with the patient, understand their condition, and treat them, the better the outcome for the patient. It could also reduce the cost of care.

24.5   Precision Medicine Is a Game Changer in Healthcare

The individualization of the treatment of diseases, called precision medicine, will open new ways for treating many diseases and break down the current way of treatment that every human is treated the same way depending on the disease. I have taken an example from my own country, Sweden, well aware of the fact that this type of healthcare is spiring and spreading at many top institutions around the world.

One-size-fits-all will be out of tune within a reasonable time: The only exception to this philosophy is for the dosing of medicines according to body weight and if you are an adult or a child.

The challenge for health providers is that an extra step in the care process comes with added cost.

The good news is that the individualization of the treatment process is likely to improve our chances to survive the disease. The most common disease to start with has been cancer. Some of the cancer drugs that are under development have a test that will let clinicians quickly diagnose if the tumor has a specific genetic twist or a specific biomarker response.[1]

Reference List, Chapter 24

1 https://news.ki.se/precision-medicine-cutting-edge-healthcare

25

CONCLUSIONS AND SUMMARY

Our society has come a long way from the early steps following the Big Bang 2,5 million years ago till today's rather well-organized society. It is a fascinating journey and unfortunately we don't know very much about the medical history from the early times called prehistoric. It is slightly easier to follow the stepwise and continued developments from the ancient medicine and onwards. The developments have gone through many learnings from pure superstition and beliefs to become more and more based on facts and proof. Different religions have had a major impact through the centuries. Sometimes not so positive or easy to live with for the general population, but despite this, it is important for our progress and it is a part of our history. There have been many bright individuals involved that have contributed with new and important ideas and knowledge, which has meant quantum leaps for humanity. Hopefully, I have managed to name and credit most of these people.

The developments in healthcare and also more generally speaking will never stop. It is against human nature. It is in our DNA to strive forward whatever discipline we are acting in. Today, we are very keen to have proof and see the effects of all medical care. This theory and principle was started by Hippocrates and is very important for the long-term progress of medicine. Today we call this *Evidence-Based Medicine*. During the days of Hippocrates, it was not easy as the effects of treatment were not always easy to interpret with the tools and knowledge of the time. The fact that these medical doctors tried to follow the rules of proven results and accurate documentation were a key to the developments that were done. Evidence-based medicine is still a challenge today and will continue to be so. It is despite the challenges, a very important principle to follow.

In modern medicine and medical technology developments it is often difficult to receive funding as the things we want to invest in today will most likely give results only for future generations. It is a classic example that many of the new ideas we would like to start today we will not see the benefit of until decades ahead. On the other hand, if we do not invest in long-term projects, it could become very expensive on the road ahead.

DOI: 10.1201/9781003393320-29

Figure 25.1   Looking for the future through binoculars will not help...

It would be fantastic if we could look into the future, but seriously we cannot even know what is coming in a day or two. What we can do, and must do, is to carefully look at the present accomplishments within technology and medicine and project how these can develop as we move forward. When we look at progress we need to consider both benefits and risks.

In my opinion the key principle to follow is what we call *Evidence-Based Technology & Medicine. Only evidence-based healthcare* can serve as a foundation to build upon and to continue the present ongoing developments and cultivate these into the future.

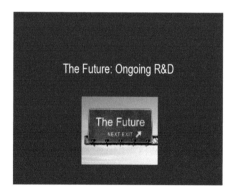

Figure 25.2   The future is often closer in time than we think...

Sometimes when we talk about the future, our perception is that it is something rather distant in time. In fact, with the higher and higher momentum of ongoing research, the future can be rather close in time.

This also means that the things we develop today also become history rather rapidly. The pace cannot be too high though, as we must obey the rule of *evidence-based medicine.* Moving too fast could result in methods and medicines that could become harmful to patients. This important fact is valid both for technology and medicine.

Two examples of medicine and methods under development:

1 In my life time, cancer has gone from being a very deadly disease (1970s and 1980s) to a disease where we are able to cure approximately 60–65% of the cases. Moreover, the research continues to move fast forward and there is a realistic hope that most types of cancer can become curable with targeted therapeutic methods, minimizing unwanted side effects.
2 Not too many years ago, we felt that a cure for Alzheimer's disease (AD) was very futuristic and not very realistic. In 2023, a new drug has received FDA approval in the United States and is also awaiting release in Europe. It is not yet a cure but will give AD patients another 2–3 years without symptoms.

Probably, the fact that we are able to diagnose AD via a simple blood test or a urine test is a key factor so that the diagnosis can be established in a practical way and early enough for patients to live longer with a meaningful life situation. There is no doubt that the new diagnostic and therapeutic methods for AD are breakthroughs that will have an impact on life quality for many patients and their families onwards. Will we be able to cure Alzheimer's disease in the future?

The cost of these medicines could be high and as such a hampering factor, and as such a challenge for society and maybe also for the individual patient.

Personally, I am convinced we will be able to find a cure for most of the neurodegenerative diseases. How quickly or when we will reach this point is impossible to guess though.

What about our future health, healthcare, medicine, and technology?

Life Expectancy Is Increasing

Within this millennium it is very likely that many persons will live until 125 years of age or longer. As a consequence, we will need to work longer and the future retirement age will be considerably higher. Maybe our retirement age will be as high as 90–100 years of age.

In many countries this will be a huge political challenge.

Remember the protests in France in the spring of 2023, when the president forced the retirement age from 62 to 64 years of age. The positive side of things ahead of us, is that we will work less with things that harm our body. Robots and artificial intelligence will take care of these heavy jobs.

Another change that most likely will need to be stimulated and increased, is *preventive medicine and care*. It will be a demand on everybody to do what is needed to stay in good shape through exercise, strength training, and healthy living and eating food that is good for your body. All of this because no healthcare system will be able to carry the workload and the cost unless we all contribute and take personal responsibility for an important part of our day to day, healthy living.

A World without Diseases – Science Fiction or Reality?

This was the title of a Swedish bioscience event in November 2022. It is a yearly event and the one in 2022 was the 10th one covering many of the new developments that have occurred during the last few years in the field of cancer, neurodegeneration, and also around Neanderthal DNA, for which, Svante Päbo received the Nobel Price, in December 2022.

In my view, the title of the event was well chosen as it is a relevant question right now as my assessment is that we have passed the science fiction stage and are entering into the reality phase.

Let's dig in and see if you agree.

Many of the challenging diseases we are focusing on today, will be curable within the next 30–50 years.

Cancer: We are today able to cure many more cancers than we were able to just 50 years ago.

Generally, the trend is good, but still some types of cancer are hard to find ways to cure. Examples of challenging types of cancer include: Lung and bronchus cancers, colorectal cancer, and pancreatic cancer. These cancers all have low survival data. One reason is that they normally are diagnosed rather late and hence challenging to cure.

Treatment methods that are showing positive results and that are being pursued with animal studies and now also being tested on humans are Immuno-therapy and Car-T treatment. In parallel, many new sensitive and specific diagnostic methods are being developed in order to diagnose cancer early and before any symptoms arise. Early detection is today the most important parameter for making it possible to treat and be cured from the cancer.

Cardiovascular disease, CVD: The most common types are, coronary heart disease, stroke, peripheral arterial disease, aortic disease. The most common reason for CVD, is build-up of fatty deposits inside the arteries (arthrosclerosis) and an increased risk of blood clots. Living a healthy life style can therefore reduce the risk of CVD. Potentially, an excellent preventive medicine method includes physical activity. For CVD, we have a large battery of diagnostic and therapeutic tools in order to save and keep people going even after an acute event. We also have tests for being able to diagnose issues early and to avoid acute situations. When it comes to CVD, we have maybe the best potential to be proactive in order to prevent the disease. Our lifestyle is mission critical and the ticking bomb I have mentioned earlier, namely *obesity* is a thing we need to avoid.

The alarming recent forecast, "Half of world will be obese by 2035, the World Obesity Federation predicts", is rather scary though. Exciting news is the research on the *INHBE gene* that could lead to the avoidance abdominal fat, by a more favorable fat distribution. (See more details in Chapter 19.)

Neurological Diseases

A stroke occurs when something blocks blood supply to part of the brain or when a blood vessel in the brain bursts.

Stroke is a disease that can be life-threatening or create severe handicap even if you fail to get care rapidly after the event. There are several risk factors for stroke and several things we can do to minimize the risk. Avoid high blood pressure/hypertension, and abandon smoking. Physical inactivity and obesity are other factors that increase the risk for a stroke. For more details, see Chapter 20.

Among the neurodegenerative diseases, *Alzheimer's disease, AD* is the most well-known. It is a devastating disease for the patient but also for the whole family. A lot of research is ongoing to find medicine and to understand the disease mechanisms. Recently, the first drug for AD was approved by the FDA, in the United States. The new drug *Lecanemab,* will "only" slow down the cognitive decline by approximately 27%.

The goal is of course to reach 100%, but remember that it is the first drug that shows a positive outcome in Alzheimer's disease so it is a good start. Medicine against AD and other neurological diseases are a must as the risk for neurodegenerative diseases increases with age, and we are living longer and longer.

Other neurological diseases where scientists are working intensely to develop treatment for are *Parkinson's disease* and *ALS (amyotrophic lateral sclerosis or Lou Gehrig's Disease)*, a rare neurological disease that affects motor neurons—those nerve cells in the brain and spinal cord that control voluntary muscle movement. More information can be found in Chapter 20.

Almost all body parts, that need repair or a replacement are today possible to replace. Organs that need replacement can in many cases be reconstructed via regenerative medicine and stem cell implementation today.

Regenerative medicine is a growing discipline and it is expected to continue to grow.

The brain will be the major challenge to replace or repair. I am not sure that our personalities will want to move to a new body.

One rather severe challenge in our society is that many of the needed long-term research investments will not benefit the present politicians, but will unfortunately only benefit the next generation of politicians and patients.

Let's hope that the politicians/governments deciding on research budgets also are visionary enough to think long term, and beyond their own political careers, for important long-term investments.

For the healthcare field in general we are on a positive trend, being able to make people live longer and in good shape.

The main challenges ahead are in my view, coming from the Climate Change, Wars, and Politics. These issues are for a totally different story…

Thanks, and Goodbye for now…

Bengt Nielsen

Communication welcome through e-mail, *nielseninnovation@gmail.com*

INDEX

Note: Page numbers in *italic* indicate a figure.

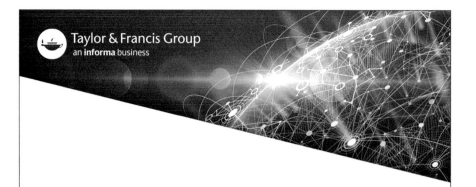